CW01472213

To the
Third Age
and **Beyond**

Preparing for retirement and growing older

Earle Wilson

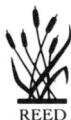

REED

REED PUBLISHING (NZ) LTD
TE KARUHI TĀ TĀPUI O REED (AOTEAROA)

Established in 1907, Reed is New Zealand's largest
book publisher, with over 600 titles in print.

www.reed.co.nz

Published by Reed Books, a division of Reed Publishing (NZ) Ltd,
39 Rawene Rd, Birkenhead, Auckland. Associated companies, branches
and representatives throughout the world.

National Library of New Zealand Cataloguing-in-Publication Data
Wilson, E. W. (Earle Wilson), 1935-
To the third age and beyond : preparing for retirement
and growing older / by Earle Wilson.
ISBN-13: 978-0-7900-1051-9
ISBN-10: 0-7900-1051-8
1. Retirement—Planning. 2. Retirees—Life skills guides.
3. Older people—Life skills guides. I. Title.
646.79—dc 22

ISBN-13: 978 0 7900 1051 9
ISBN-10: 0 7900 1051 8

Text illustrations by Richard Gunther
Cover design and illustration by Cathy Bignell

Printed in China

Contents

For Jenni, together with whom
I continue to grow

Introduction

This book has been written primarily for people approaching retirement and their families, although much of it also concerns people who have already retired and are starting to face the prospect of growing older. My principal reason for writing this book is the number of people with whom I have come into contact, or heard about, who have either clearly made wrong choices at the time of retirement or failed to prepare themselves adequately for this important life step and the steps that follow.

A second reason is that there are many families with old and often frail parents who do not know where to start when some solutions are needed for the care of these people.

Another reason is that a demographic shift in the population is about to hit — in some countries it is already hitting — the developed world. This shift has been called 'global ageing' and comes with the baby-boomer generation. These people are starting to reach their late fifties and in the near future will form a powerful group both economically and politically. Future governments may tremble at the thought of the grey vote. There are now examples of two generations in retirement and soon there may even be a third. These are the people for whom much of this book has been written.

The third age
The expectation seems to have been that once retired one did nothing much of importance — a little gardening perhaps, and games of cards with friends — filling in time

until infirmity and death came along. No longer. Although the great majority of people at some time will give up working, and all will grow older, the word 'retirement' itself also has become outdated. *Le troisième âge* is a phrase used by the French to describe the age that follows the rearing of a family and a life in work or business. We'll just call it the third age and I think it is a more apt phrase to use in the twenty-first century. This is because what used to be thought of as retirement is now much more of a transition from one lifestyle to another: some sort of work may continue. It is the way you live your life that will change. You can also think of it as yet another chance to do those things you have always wanted to do.

Retirement in the past

There was a time when it was accepted that employees, whatever industry they were in, would reach a retirement age and then stop work, sometimes rewarded with a gold watch. While some employers may have deliberately, or even unwittingly, pushed people towards retirement in order to get rid of them, some employees, usually those with separate interests or skills, have found themselves pulled towards retirement and the prospect of a new life. The retirement age has gradually crept up over the years and now stands conventionally, but not compulsorily, at 65.

Ageism

Ageism is a term that recently has surfaced to describe discrimination against older people, perhaps those over 55 or so, in the belief that they are no longer useful or competent members of society. This belief can affect older people to the extent that they accept it themselves. Let us be quite clear about this, *old is not dumb* and *old is not useless.*

These are guiding principles in this book and they should be inscribed in burning letters on the desk of every human resources manager.

The fateful Monday morning

At some stage most people will give up work voluntarily, some will be made redundant, others will just wear out! Whatever the reason, on some fateful Monday morning you will not be going to work, or possibly you will be going off to do something different. The pattern of life will have to change, the daily routine will be different. Now you will have the time to do all those things you have always wanted to do; that is, if you know what they are! Now you will be able to wear what you like, eat when you want to, read the newspaper, watch television, listen to the radio, go for a drive. How boring. Do you *really* want to do that every day? Seven days a week? Of course not. The third age is not about being on holiday.

The third age is also not about giving up; it *is* about doing something different with your life. It is also about continuing to grow. But doing something different with your life is not the kind of thing you can just stumble into; it needs preparation. You need to work at it, perhaps over a few years. It is my belief that this book will help you through that process of preparing and planning.

This is not another book about financial planning; there are plenty of those around, some better than others. Of course, the financial side of things does need to be planned and some aspects of financial planning are included here. But mostly this is a book about all the other things you need to plan: where to live, what sort of home, health matters, activities, clubs and societies, living in a new community; all, or most, of the details people seem not to think about.

Relationships

Relationships also may change when you reach the third age. I know of more than one instance when, on the fateful Monday morning, the wife, who has her own routine, her own friends, her own schedule, has been confronted by this pathetic figure asking what he should do now. It becomes worse. The wife wants to go out for coffee with the girls; he wants to go too and has to be told, 'No way'. And so it goes on, day after day: 'What can I do now?', 'Can I help you?', 'What'll we do today?' It is a sorry story, but one that is all too frequently repeated. Relationships with other family members and with friends can also change.

What happens next?

The third age, or retirement if you still prefer it, is not the end. It is the beginning of another chapter in your life; it is not the final chapter and you need to think about the fourth and even fifth ages. Possibly you will plan to buy a lifestyle block and grow grapes or olives, or raise a few sheep. Great, but there will come a day when the work gets a bit too much and the property becomes a chore rather than a delight. Time to start another planned chapter. We can spend a good ten years doing one thing and when that becomes too difficult move on to doing something else. All planned for in outline, not necessarily in detail, for the detail may have to change to suit financial or physical circumstances.

Growing older

Growing older also needs a bit of preparation. Why? Because one day you will not be able to do all the things you can do now and there will be time freed up to do other things. Also, there will be health problems to face, maybe your partner to look after when he or she becomes sick or frailer than you are yourself. How will you deal with all this if you haven't thought ahead? The answer is — badly!

So a part of this book considers preparing for growing old and growing even older; growing old and staying as well as possible. Even if you do have a few health problems, when someone asks, 'How are you?' you want to be able to say, 'I'm very well, thank you'. It is hoped that some of the advice in these pages will help you to keep saying that for many, many years.

Everything in these pages applies equally to women and to men, or the other way around. In those one or two instances where there may be gender differences they are mentioned. Although there are many references to partners I hope that single people, and there are many in the third and following ages, will find that most, if not all, of what has been written applies equally to them.

Old is not dumb; old is not useless

Throughout I have tried to maintain several themes:

▷ Successful retirement and healthy ageing are all about having a positive attitude.

▷ Just because you are old you are not stupid or incompetent: *old is not dumb* and *old is not useless*.

▷ Preparing and planning can save you from mistakes.

▷ You should *continue to grow* for as long as possible.

▷ Living alone should not mean that you are lonely.

I hope you will enjoy the third age as much as I do and that you will look forward to the ages still to come.

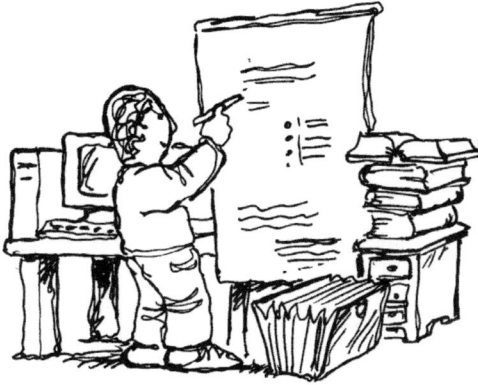

1

Getting started

Planning and planners

Preparation for retirement usually starts during the years leading up to ending full-time work. Ideally, it should start as soon as you start work but being realistic it will start much later. In what follows some aspects of the planning process are described in outline. No one can provide you with a template for planning for the third age — everyone's dreams and needs are different.

Planning is a process whereby goals, or objectives, are defined and strategies to reach those goals are formulated. That is a rather formal statement, but it does distinguish between what your dreams are and how you are going to reach them. Not everyone is good at planning; in fact, most of us are probably quite poor at it! However, that should not prevent us from trying to plan, as in the trying we may well come up against a whole lot of things we never thought of.

People and planning

People can be divided into three categories. Those who are:

 ▷ detailed planners

 ▷ general planners

 ▷ vague dreamers.

Detailed planners emerge more frequently the closer people get to actual retirement. However, some individuals are by nature detailed planners who, while planning everything meticulously, may be blind to alternatives when circumstances change. General planners concentrate on the bigger picture and leave room for variation while preserving an overall scheme. Vague dreamers generally allow events to overtake them and unaided they don't actually plan many things themselves. They may be given to wild and unpractical schemes and need to be held in check. They can be changed but they are unlikely to become detailed planners.

Varieties of planning

Planning can be:

 ▷ short term, meaning monthly or weekly

 ▷ medium term, often defined more by social events such as marriage or graduation than by clock time

 ▷ long term, well into the future.

Planning also can be:

 ▷ active or passive

 ▷ anticipatory and positive

▷ precautionary and negative.

Planning is influenced by age and gender as well as educational background and personal economic situation. Add to all of this financial planning and lifestyle planning and you can understand that the whole business requires a lot of thought. There is good evidence that people who are in relatively lowly paid work are least likely to plan for retirement, yet these are just the people who probably most need that planning.

When to start

In an ideal situation, planning for the third age should start as soon as one enters the work force, which usually will be in the early to mid twenties, or even before. But to be realistic, most people will be likely to place other, and more immediate, goals higher in priority than retirement; marriage, career, children, a first home are all likely to take priority. Nevertheless, while it may not be possible to define one's retirement goals with any precision, the need to have sufficient money for retirement should be obvious. With this in mind the importance of starting some kind of savings scheme is important when you join the workforce. Added to this is the fact that many people underestimate the age to which they will live and leave themselves short. A few dollars saved on a regular basis will eventually grow to a worthwhile amount. There is more about this in the financial planning section (chapter 9).

Be positive

Planning, as with so many things to do with retirement, depends on attitude. Start with a negative attitude, one that regards retirement as the end of the line, a sort of waiting for death, and that is exactly what you will do and what will happen. Start with the attitude that retirement is the start of a new chapter in your life and that is just what you will be able to achieve. Without that positive 'I am going to do something' attitude, planning becomes an empty and pointless exercise and probably will not even happen.

Do not be put off by the word planning. Many people will shudder and say, 'I don't know where to begin', not knowing how to start or what to do next. You do not need a pencil and paper, or even a fancy software program; just sit down and think what your objectives might be. Once you have decided those it is time to think how you are going to reach them.

This is the point at which you can do a SWOT analysis. Decide your:

▷ **S**trengths

▷ **W**eaknesses

▷ **O**pportunities

▷ **T**hreats.

Thinking in this way helps focus your thoughts and attack the whole planning thing better. Talk it over with someone you trust. Ask them about your strengths and weaknesses because different opinions are sometimes helpful. What are the opportunities for you to meet your objectives? Fish farming is difficult if you live in a desert. What are the threats, the obstacles?

Strategies

Often the objectives themselves help decide the strategy. If you want to have a pig farm you will need to look for suitable land, not a mid-city apartment. Once the objectives have been thought out they should be turned over, thought through again, and alternatives considered. Are you being too ambitious? Do you have too many objectives? Can you meet even half of them? It is sensible to err on the side of too few objectives rather than too many; you probably will not need more than three or four. Now you can begin to plan your strategies for each of these objectives in more detail.

Below is a sample of what you might come up with supposing you had set yourself three objectives:

1. To grow and process my own olives and market the product.

2. To have a six-month world trip.

3. To take up playing bowls.

Clearly, the first of these is the one that will take the most planning and may even need a pencil and paper. There are actually three objectives here: grow the olives, process them and market the result. The other two objectives also need strategies but they are much simpler. So looking at the first objective the strategies might include:

▷ research the subject and talk with experts

▷ select and purchase suitable land and tractor

▷ purchase suitable variety of olives

▷ plant olives

▷ build processing shed

▷ purchase olive press, sorting tables, harvesting gear, pruning gear, oil containers

▷ research market for oil.

One could go on in ever increasing detail because each of these is an objective in itself and requires its own strategies, but it is an outline of the things that will be needed to be achieved if the primary objective is to be met.

The second objective is much more short term and, on the surface at least, easier to plan. But here, too, one does need to get everything sorted. For example:

▷ decide on which countries to visit

▷ work out how long in each place

▷ decide how to travel — sea or air

▷ choose an agent if you decide not to do the booking yourself

▷ take advice

▷ get passports

▷ get travel insurance

▷ choose cruise lines/airlines

▷ arrange money

▷ arrange for someone to take care of things while you are away (power of attorney).

As with all such lists the detail can turn out to be formidable, but break it all down and it becomes much easier to plan.

The third objective, learning to play bowls, is the easiest:

▷ get in touch with a club

▷ arrange to have some sort of instruction

▷ join the club

▷ buy a set of bowls and the right clothes

▷ go for it!

Alternatively, discover after giving it a try that you didn't like it or showed no aptitude and decide to learn to play croquet instead. All these things have in common a set of strategies that allow you to meet your objectives.

Beyond the third age

The kind of planning needed for growing older is different, in that it is not so easy to clearly define the goals. The overall goal, of course, is to remain as well as possible for as long as possible, but the illnesses/disabilities that may occur are not predictable. What is needed is an overall scheme of what will happen if either you or your partner suffer some sort of setback. Apart from the knotty question of asset testing if residential care is needed, which it will not be in the great majority of cases, financial planning is less important than planning for a creakier lifestyle. Such planning should be positive and never negative; attitude is all important and *old is not dumb*.

While it will not be possible to plan for every possible crisis, an overall scheme should be thought through and discussed with your partner and your family well ahead of any major health problem. People sometimes panic when faced with a health incident, such as a stroke or heart attack, and make wrong decisions. It is better for everyone to have in mind a general plan so that you, your partner and particularly your family know what you or they are going to do, if anything.

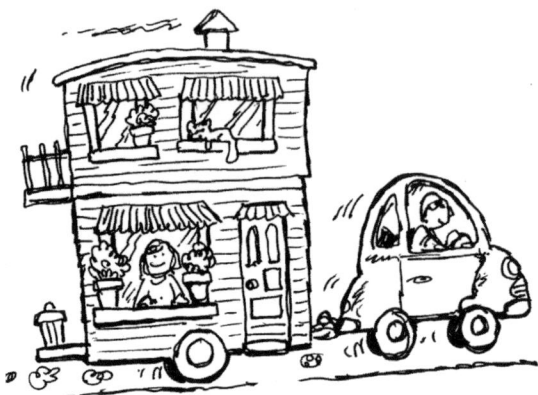

2

Size matters

Where to live

Preparing for retirement has to include the central decision of where you are going to live. This in turn depends on what you want to do, what your partner wants to do, how you both are going to spend your time and how old you are. It is hard to rear prize sheep in a city, and impractical to go often to the theatre when you live 100 kilometres away. The decision also is linked to ageing: a house in the country might be fine for a few years but may not suit when age starts to take over.

There can be no hard and fast rules about this decision, each person or couple have to make their own, possibly unique, decision. So, what are the options? Here are a few to think about:

    ▷ stay where you are

▷ move to an apartment

▷ go to the beach

▷ buy a lifestyle block

▷ become modern gypsies

▷ live near the family

▷ downsize your home

▷ buy into a retirement village

▷ move into an Abbeyfield house

▷ go into a rest home.

Stay where you are

It is quite possible you want to stay in the house you've lived in for the last 30 or 40 years, but this does not suit everyone. For some people staying where they have lived for a long time is the best decision. They may be comfortable in a particular neighbourhood, have a number of close friends, and belong to clubs and societies in the area. Such people should have some very good reason for wanting to live somewhere else.

A woman, now in her seventies, has lived in the same house in a smaller city for 35 years. She has three daughters, all married, living within a few blocks. She and her husband, when he was retiring, consciously decided to stay where they were. He has since died and, although alone, she is perfectly happy knowing she has family support nearby. The family look after the property and she will continue to live there for as long as possible.

Move to an apartment

What about an apartment? It could be an ideal choice. The advantages of many modern apartment blocks include:

▷ no maintenance worries

▷ security, especially when you take long holidays or travel abroad

▷ secure covered parking

▷ in some cases, leisure facilities such as a pool or gymnasium.

It is not quite that easy, though. Most apartment blocks have a body corporate responsible for maintenance of the building and communal areas as well as rates, insurance and the rest. You will be paying a contribution to all this.

Size matters: there needs to be sufficient room for each of you to have your own space and this can be made more difficult with an open-plan layout. Make sure that the apartment is adequately sound proofed. Noisy sound systems or gurgling plumbing can be a nightmare. Check all these things out before you move in.

Also, if you enjoy a spot of gardening think very carefully before choosing an apartment unless you have a spacious deck or balcony. 'Oh, we'll have a small place in the country as well; we can garden there.' Which one will be home? You will find yourself endlessly travelling between one place and the other if you do not plan carefully and think about the pitfalls. Another problem with the second home is the need to go there rather than anywhere else when you are having a longer spell away; the second home can become a tie.

Things to consider when thinking of moving into an apartment:

▷ Find out about the body corporate — who runs it, who makes the decisions, and what the annual payments are.

▷ If you are used to the great outdoors, think again.

▷ Keen on pets? Think again.

Go to the beach

What about the holiday house or bach (crib) that you have always thought you might retire to one day? Perhaps do it up a bit and improve the facilities. It sounds enticing and maybe it is; perhaps it is your ideal. But be careful that the holiday home doesn't become a prison when you discover after a few months that you've nothing to occupy your time. The neighbours you get on so well with are only there sometimes and most of the other holiday homes in the area are also vacant. The place is empty; nothing to do, stuck miles away from anywhere much and winter is approaching. Still sound attractive?

A variant of this is to move to a holiday resort area such as Queenstown or the Bay of Islands or Taupo. Be careful: property is not cheap in these places and they are relatively isolated from major services, particularly health facilities. However, the climate is good, there are plenty of things to do and there are many people of a similar age.

A couple decided to retire after the husband had several heart attacks and his condition wasn't suitable for surgery. They lived in a small North Island city and decided to move to Wanaka for the fishing. They bought a property on a fairly steep section, neither of them being gardeners, and soon discovered that managing on the steep slope wasn't easy.

Would you make the same mistake: move away from expert medical care and take on something for which you are physically not suitable?

Buy a lifestyle block

Many so-called lifestyle blocks are too small to generate a reasonable income and too large to look after properly if you don't graze an area or plant useful crops. Probably 4 hectares (about 10 acres) is the least area that can provide you with any useful income. However, there is no point in buying any such block unless you have a clear idea of the use you are going to make of the land. Decide what you want and remember that one day you will probably have to move to a smaller property.

For obvious reasons most lifestyle blocks are in rural or semi-rural areas, which means that there is a degree of isolation from neighbours and from shopping. Is this what you want? Whoever is doing the heavy work, and there will be heavy work, needs to consider the other partner. Will they feel the isolation? Will they be bored? Are you both in the whole thing together or is the enterprise for the gratification of one person only?

If you do decide to go the lifestyle way make sure that you try and become part of the local community by joining sporting or social clubs or societies. You are not just buying a lifestyle property; you are moving into a living community that can offer you a lot and to which you should have an obligation.

Become modern gypsies

The people who buy or build motor-homes or, less commonly, caravans and take off travelling the country permanently probably will object to me calling them gypsies but the lifestyles are similar. There are a number of couples and probably single people as well who sell up, buy a motor-home and take to the road. Fine: a very good and enjoyable way to see the country and meet a variety of people, some of them also in motor-homes doing the same thing. There also are people who set off on an extended cruise in their own yacht, which is a similar choice.

But this lifestyle cannot be anything but temporary, for there comes a point when it is necessary to go back to living in a house or equivalent. Be careful.

Fred and Judy, both in their late sixties, sold their suburban three-bedroom house and section and bought a motor-home. For two years they had a wonderful time travelling around the country, sometimes stopping in one place for a couple of months. They went to several motor-home rallies and met lots of new people. Then Judy became ill. While her condition was not life threatening, it did mean they would have to give up travelling. So, they decided to sell the motor-home and buy a house in a small town that was still close enough to a city. Reality struck: there was barely enough money left from the sale of their former house and the motor-home had depreciated far more than they expected. They could not afford to buy to the standard they had previously enjoyed.

If you make this choice be sure that you have enough capital earning as much interest as possible during your time in the motor-home or afloat. Fred and Judy probably should have thought about saving up for the motor-home and renting out their house while they were away.

Live near the family

Think very carefully before you consider moving closer to your family, a move often associated with downsizing. It is nice to think that moving closer to the children will somehow benefit both groups. Sometimes it certainly does, but often it results in family tensions that simply would not exist if there was some distance between you. Nothing is worse than having your mother-in-law, son-in-law, daughter, whomever, call at the house *every* day. And when the expected baby-sitting service breaks down for whatever reason, children dumped on granddad and grandma four times a week can become a bit much very quickly. It really is much better to remain at some distance. Anyway, with present-day mobility what do you do when the children decide to go and live somewhere else? Go with them?

Downsize your home

Downsizing is a common thought. Why not realise some of the capital tied up in the over-large house you own, move to something smaller and invest what's left over to provide additional income? For some this may be a very realistic option and one that deserves serious consideration. But *size matters*. If you decide to downsize and end up with only one or two bedrooms, you need to think about where the family will stay when they want to spend some time with you. Suppose you have two married children and grandchildren: they will not want the extra expense of staying in a motel around the corner or the discomfort of a tent in the garden. They will stop visiting; it has been known to happen. If you wish to see them you will have to go to them. And will you have room for the grandchildren to come and stay? A good choice might be to downsize from a large property to a moderate-sized house on a smaller section.

The success or otherwise of this step often can depend on where the move is to and what type of accommodation is moved into — townhouse, apartment, smaller house — everyone will have a different idea. Just make sure you are making the decision that will be right for you for at least the next ten years. If family live in the same general area this may be a very sensible move. They can still come and visit you without the need to stay over.

Capital released by downsizing can have several benefits. Some overseas travel may be funded. Certainly a top-up of available income comes in handy and may even be needed to offset the rising cost of health insurance, remembering that this will go up with increasing age.

Housing in the fourth and fifth ages

Take action ahead of the need

As you become even older the biggest decision you will have to make will be about housing:

  ▷ Is the present house too big and the garden too
     much trouble?

  ▷   If the house is still suitable, does it need a bit
     of alteration to make access easier?

  ▷ Can the garden be redesigned to make it easy care
     or even no care?

  ▷ Is the interior lighting adequate for comfortable
     reading?

  ▷ Are all the appliances easily operated and not too
     heavy?

  ▷ Has the potential for falls been minimised; are the

floors slippery? Are there mats or rugs that might trip people?

▷ Are the steps too steep?

▷ Are falls a problem in icy or wet weather?

▷ Can you walk to the shops?

▷ What will happen when you can no longer drive your car?

▷ Is it time to consider a retirement village or similar?

Inability to drive a car is often a huge problem for some people, particularly those who do not live close to public transport. Many people will be affected by failure of eyesight or other health issues that render them unfit to possess a licence to drive. The situation is made doubly worse if the partner is a driver who has either lost confidence or also doesn't have a licence.

As people grow older losing their driving licence is the largest worry of all. Perhaps this event really does signal a need for a change of housing: somewhere smaller and on a bus route, or close to one; an apartment or townhouse; at least somewhere with a smaller garden.

Better to have made that move ahead of the need. And this is the key to planning for the ageing process: *take action ahead of the need*. Do not wait for severe arthritis, heart problems or perhaps a stroke to make it obvious that something has to change. Some conditions, such as arthritis, give a warning of what may be to come. Use that warning. Anticipate and make the changes in your lifestyle before you face a crisis. Sooner or later there will almost certainly be a crisis of some kind.

For a lot of people, staying in their own home is what they would prefer, and many manage very well. They may be eligible for home help. This is a service for people with a disability or for the frail elderly. Depending on the need, which is determined by a formal needs assessment undertaken by the local district health board, you may be entitled to help with housework, washing, showering and so on. You may be entitled to receive meals on wheels, too. The assistance available, which also can be privately purchased, enables people to stay in the place they know rather than enter a rest home.

Buy into a retirement village

Increasingly, retirement villages are being advertised, often in a very enticing way, as an ideal solution to retirement living. If you are fit, active and enjoy the company of younger people it is probably not for you; not yet, anyway. In a survey conducted by the University of Otago the average age of residents in the retirement villages surveyed was 79.9 years, and most of the residents, 68 percent, were women. However, more and more the retirement village industry is directing its efforts to much younger age groups, even to those barely over 50, with a number of lifestyle options. This trend is being seen overseas also: in Australia, South Africa and the United States large complexes with varied leisure facilities are on offer. As the baby-boomers come through into their middle or late fifties the same thing is happening here. Before you consider this option you do need to ask yourself whether you want to spend all your time in a fairly restricted community that has no young people.

Accommodation varies from individual villas with up to three bedrooms to townhouses or even serviced apartments. Some villages have a rest home on the same site, or even a hospital as well. This means that you can move through the various levels of care as needed.

There is no doubt that the retirement village concept is an attractive one for those who no longer wish to be bothered with keeping up a large garden or house. There can be potential social benefits as well. Most villages have communal facilities and many have recreational facilities as well, so there can be opportunities for residents to meet and interact. What is less clear is the extent to which residents actually make use of these opportunities and, sadly, there can be many lonely people in retirement villages. Nevertheless, most people seem to expect they will have a more enjoyable time in a village. There is a weekly or monthly charge for maintenance of the property and communal facilities, including insurance. All villages have some sort of management structure. Management has final authority over the concern and it may or may not take into consideration suggestions or requests from a residents' committee.

Occupation options

The ownership structure also is an important consideration. The common ones are:

▷ licence to occupy

▷ lifetime lease

▷ unit title

▷ cross-lease.

Most villages operate on the licence-to-occupy system whereby residents purchase the right to live in a particular house for the rest of their lives. On leaving the unit the licence is sold on, usually to the owners of the village.

Here there are potential pitfalls in that any capital gain on the licence will not necessarily accrue to the occupant. Most villages operating under this system have a statutory supervisor, usually a trustee company, that looks after residents' rights. Other options include: outright ownership of the unit; registered lifetime interest, giving an interest on the land owned by the village; unit title with fees paid to a body corporate or a manager; cross-lease, with all the land owned jointly and a lease from the joint ownership to the individual owner/s; freehold title, with fees paid as above.

Safeguards and standards

The Retirement Villages Association (see 'Want more?', page 124) has a code of practice and minimum operating standards that cover the financial information that must be supplied to residents, termination of contracts, privacy matters and so on. In addition, all member villages must have a disputes resolution process, with anything that cannot be resolved on site being referred to the association's own review authority. Listed villages are graded as full members or probationary members in the process of undergoing audit to see whether or not they comply with the association's standards.

The *Retirement Villages Act*, which is due to come into force in March 2006, will require all retirement villages to be registered and to have a statutory supervisor. In addition there will be a code of practice that will require full disclosure of certain key information before a prospective resident signs an occupation agreement. There has to be a facility for dealing with complaints and a formal disputes resolution procedure. The Act contains detailed provisions covering the period before a prospective resident enters the village, during the period of occupation and after the resident leaves the facility.

Check it out thoroughly

Anyone contemplating buying into a retirement village really does need to examine the fine print very carefully and get answers to a number of questions, some of which are listed below. But before that you should check whether the village has the following facilities:

- ▷ full maintenance of gardens and units

- ▷ security patrols

- ▷ emergency call system

- ▷ 24-hour assistance

- ▷ communal centre

- ▷ recreational facilities

- ▷ services such as hairdressing

- ▷ a rest home.

Once you are satisfied that the village has everything you may want there are the other questions:

- ▷ Is the location where you want to be?

- ▷ Remembering that *size matters*: is your prospective unit big enough?

- ▷ What leisure facilities are there?

- ▷ Is transport available?

- ▷ What say can you have in the running of the village?

- ▷ What are the ongoing fees and what do they cover?

- ▷ Are there additional one-off charges and what are they for?

▷ Are there guarantees if the business is sold?

▷ What is the track record of the managers? Do they run other similar organisations successfully?

▷ Is management sensitive to the needs of older people?

▷ What happens if you want or have to leave, and how much of your investment do you get back?

It may be that the village you are considering is under development and you have the chance to buy off the plans. These are some of the additional questions:

▷ Have the developers done this kind of thing before and were they successful?

▷ How is the project financed?

▷ Can the developers deliver on their promises and on time?

▷ How and by whom is any money you pay in advance held?

▷ Will you be repaid in full if the project folds?

▷ Will the developers be involved in management of the village and, if not, who will manage it?

These questions are not exhaustive and it is imperative that anyone thinking seriously about purchasing a unit in a retirement village should seek the services of a lawyer experienced in property matters. Families of older people particularly need to be aware of the possible pitfalls and make sure that their parents or grandparents get the best possible legal advice.

Move to an Abbeyfield house

Another option for the single elderly person seeking a more social existence is one of the houses run by the Abbeyfield Society. There are now several of these houses around the country.

Abbeyfield houses can be thought of as flatting for the elderly but with a few extras, such as cooked meals. A typical Abbeyfield house has about ten residents, both men and women, each with their own spacious bedroom/sitting room and bathroom. These rooms are furnished and maintained by the residents themselves. Two meals a day are provided by a live-in housekeeper in a communal dining area, and there are other communal areas. The cost of living in an Abbeyfield house can normally be met by New Zealand superannuation plus a housing allowance. For most of these houses there is a waiting list.

An Abbeyfield house is ideal for the lonely, single elderly. It is not a rest home and residents can be largely self-sufficient. Often, families can stay over in a suite reserved for this purpose. This suite also can be used for a trial stay so the prospective resident and those already resident can assess each other.

Go into a rest home

Although at any one time only about 4 percent of those over the age of 65 are residents of a rest home or residential care facility, a much higher percentage, perhaps as many as 30 percent, of people over the age of 65 will spend some of their life in such a facility. Some rest homes may provide a kind of transition service between hospital and home, particularly for stroke victims, but most are simply residential care facilities for frail elderly who cannot manage or be cared for at home.

A rest home may also have geriatric hospital facilities able to care for those who are completely incapable of looking after themselves, usually those elderly who are suffering from one or another form of dementia. Admission to these facilities is usually preceded by an in-depth assessment arranged through the appropriate department of the local district health board.

Assessing needs

Entry into a rest home may be by private arrangement; that is, you or your family pay for you to be accommodated, cared for and fed. An alternative is to enter through a 'needs assessment' process operated by the local district health board (DHB). If you are judged to be incapable of living in your own home, the DHB will pay for the rest home costs subject to income and asset testing. If you have assets and/ or income over a certain amount you will be required to pay all or some part of the costs from those sources.

Choosing a rest home

There are many rest homes in New Zealand, some with names suggesting they are only one step short of the funeral director: Golden Years, Autumn Leaves. The quality of care offered by these homes can be quite variable and a few are rather dismal places, so caution is needed in selecting one suitable for yourself, your partner or an elderly relative. A useful source of reference is the Eldernet website, which provides a wealth of information on selecting a rest home as well as providing, for some areas, a list of rest homes with vacancies. Recent government legislation has tightened up the accreditation of rest homes so in the future there may be less variation in quality of care.

As with retirement villages there are questions about the facilities, training of staff, medical care and so on, that should be asked during a visit to the home. First of all decide on the locality, contact the rest homes in that area and then visit them all. Places that look wonderful from the street can feel gloomy inside. You want a place that feels happy so assessing the atmosphere is important. Take note of the availability of public transport and convenience for visiting by friends and family. Some specific questions to consider are:

▷ Is the place clean and homely?

▷ Are there social areas where residents can meet?

▷ Is there a garden where residents can walk or sit?

▷ Are the rooms attractive and well lit? Are they sunny?

▷ Can residents have their own telephone and television?

▷ Can residents have some of their own furniture and pictures?

▷ Are the meals varied, attractive and nutritious?

▷ Is there a variety of leisure facilities?

▷ Are there arranged outings? How often and to where?

▷ Are the staff well trained, respectful and understanding of older people's needs?

▷ Is there 24-hour medical cover?

▷ Can residents have their own general practitioner?

▷ Is there laughter about the place?

▷ Does the place seem to be run for the benefit of the residents or for the convenience of the staff?

The list is endless and everyone will have different things to ask about, although for me the last two questions are essential. The main message is that you must assure yourself that you are making the right choice.

Financing residential care

If a needs assessment confirms that you are in need of long-term care in a licensed rest home or hospital, you will be eligible for a residential care subsidy subject to asset and income testing. Your house is not included in assets while your partner is still living there, but is included if you both are in care. The government has signalled its intention to progressively remove asset testing, but not income testing, for those aged 65 years and over. Starting in 2005 the asset limits for a single or widowed person, or for a couple both in care, is $150,000. For a couple where one is in care the limit is $55,000 plus house and car. These limits are set to rise by $10,000 a year.

Because income testing is not being removed, if you have income from any source, including New Zealand super-annuation, you will have to pass on up to $636 a week to pay for your care. This excludes a weekly allowance of $30.06 and an annual clothing allowance of $212.89. You also may be able to retain half your income from New Zealand-registered superannuation schemes or annuities.

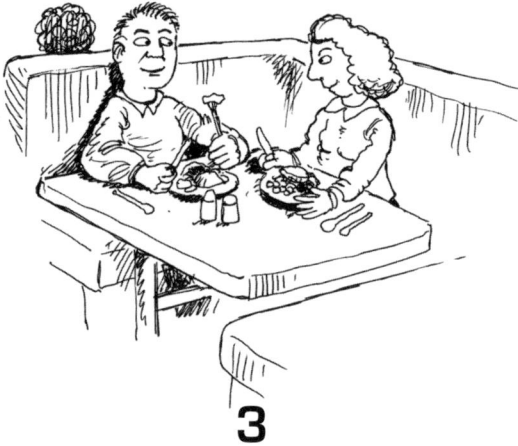

3

Who do you want to push your wheelchair?

Relationships

Almost certainly, along with the other changes in your life associated with retirement, there will be changes in your relationships: with your partner, perhaps with your children, possibly with your grandchildren, probably with your friends. These changes cannot be planned but they do need to be understood and prepared for. Some of the potential challenges may not be as easy to meet as you imagine. But most couples will find the transition to the third age enhancing for their relationship and will be rewarded by many years of happy companionship. These are people who are each other's best friends and who will be delighted to either push the wheelchair or have the other one push.

Relationship changes

It is at times of change that the best and the worst aspects of any relationship come to the surface. Retirement is one of those times of change, and it is the changing nature of your relationships that may prove the biggest challenge to you and to those around you. Sometimes relationships are strengthened by the change, such as when qualities that once were attractive become recognised again. For others, relationships may worsen and even become intolerable.

Creaking doors

Sadly, there are relationships that have creaked along for years. Many of these have been held together by a common purpose, such as the rearing of a family. Others have managed to survive because not much time is spent together, one or both being at work all day and often with separate activities in the evenings or at weekends. Little habits that for years have been tolerated may become sources of irritation, or even active dislike. Sometimes the failure of a relationship is acknowledged by at least one of the partners but the people stay together because it is thought to be too difficult, too expensive, or simply too much trouble, to face a definitive change.

If you do need to end the relationship don't mess about; just get on and do it whether you are the wife, the husband, or the de facto. There will be pain, the family may even be split, but in the long run everyone will probably be happier. Make sure that you both take legal advice and try to ensure that the process of separation and divorce, if that is to be the decision, is as straightforward as possible. Do try to avoid an acrimonious dispute with mud flying all over the place and everyone becoming thoroughly miserable and angry. Sure you may feel injured. Sure you may even feel bitter.

But remember that you have had good times. Put the pain behind you and get on with the rest of your life.

Talk together

What if one of the partners is not in the workforce but at home looking after the house, garden, children, grand-children or whatever? How does such a partner get involved in the planning for retirement process? The first thing is that it is essential in preparing for retirement that the other partner is fully involved and understands what will or will not happen, because they also have to plan for a change in their life.

Retirement is something that both partners have to do together because the rhythm of life for both of them will change, and that change may bring with it potential difficulties within the relationship. It does not need to: discuss what will happen; together think through the poss-ible pitfalls; sort it all out. Just because you are suddenly thrust into each other's company 24 hours a day does not mean that you have to be side by side constantly or talking to each other all day. Create your own spaces, not only physical but also mental.

Together all day every day

It may happen that both partners retire from the workforce at much the same time and from different jobs. For example, one may have been a nurse, the other an office worker. Suddenly, with retirement, both are taken out of the famil-iarity of their respective workplaces and condemned, or overjoyed, to spend all that time together. But it is one thing to spend weekends or holidays with each other, quite another to spend all day every day together for the rest of your lives. It is perhaps something you have never done before in your lives, at least not for any length of time. You will have to work out between you how you are going to accommodate your separate wants and needs. Try to create the opportunities for being apart. Try to develop some separate interests so that you both have an exposure to different groups of people while retaining the friends you have in common.

Create spaces

There will be many times when you both have to be in the same house together for most of the day. With planning you can establish areas within the house that you can each call your own in some way. Traditionally for a man this would probably have been the garage and a workshop, while the wife had a sewing room. This will no longer do. Now the spaces tend to overlap: the computer, for instance, or even the kitchen. Gardens can be useful spaces, but not everyone likes to garden, or can, and then there are the rainy days. Men probably lean towards vegetable growing and women more towards flowers and shrubs. This gives both their set spaces, occasional havens.

This book cannot tell you what your spaces should be, only that you should have them.

Connie and Jack both worked. Connie ran her own floristry business; Jack was a teacher. Jack took retirement at 65 and Connie decided to sell her business and join him. Although they always had worked apart they had a close relationship, liked being together and enjoyed the same things: they both played golf; and they enjoyed music, books, the theatre and good eating. But they recognised the need to have their own spaces. They spent some of the money from the sale of Connie's business on converting their house to provide separate areas in which each could be self-sufficient and shared areas where they could come together. After ten years the arrangement is still working well and they are spending more and more time in the shared space.

Continue to grow

You may think you stopped growing in your twenties, and physically you did. This is not about that kind of growing but about growing as a person. You grow through your experiences and the things you learn. You may grow in relationships; indeed, relationships have a life of their own and that means they can grow, stagnate, or even die. In the best relationships the partners continue to grow by feeding on one another, each nourishing the other by their achievements. Think about *growing* older and not just getting older.

Arrested development

We don't all continue to grow throughout our lives. Many people stop at some point, often in the forties, and never go any further as people. They stay in a kind of personality rut, their beliefs unchanging, their tastes remaining the same. Physically these people grow older but in personal terms their development has been arrested. Do not become one of these people. Your attitude should be that you are going to keep growing for as long as possible and that nothing is going to get in the way.

One tragedy that is all too common is where one partner in a relationship continues to grow and the other does not. This might spell the end of things, but often the relationship drags on with neither partner recognising the cause of the change. If you can recognise what has happened it may be possible to rekindle growth. There is usually a reason for growth stopping and finding the reason is the key to solving the situation.

Very often the reason for someone ceasing to grow and develop is that there is a loss of interest. The things that used to interest one no longer do so and there are no replacements. But there is always something that will interest a person and every effort should be made to find that something. This is when it is important to be in touch with the activities within one's community, because that is where the interest is likely to come from. It certainly will not come from the television screen.

Down in the dumps

Another cause for arrested growth and a loss of interest is mild depression, which is quite common in older people and, of course, may happen to younger people as well. There are many causes of mild depression and often this condition, which can be effectively treated, goes unrecognised. Mild depression also may be a major cause of memory loss, as well as sleep disturbance, loss of appetite, unwillingness to take exercise and so on. If you, or your partner, or your elderly relatives, develop these symptoms a visit to the doctor and the initiation of treatment will usually result in improvement.

Get in early. Do not put off the visit to the doctor hoping things will get better of their own accord. It will usually be the partner who provides the drive to see the doctor as very often the person doesn't realise, or doesn't admit, they have a problem. But for those who live alone realising there is a problem will fall upon someone else, perhaps a friend or neighbour. Do not be afraid to help if you are the friend or the neighbour.

Humour

A sense of humour is a rewarding attribute; when it is shared by your partner it is more than doubly rewarding. Couples who can and do laugh together are among the happiest people I know, and they also are people who get over difficult times quickly. So find things, even silly things, to laugh at and enjoy the fun. You will find that laughter relieves tensions and can be a powerful boost to your positive attitude.

Hearing and listening

Some couples, although they hear each other, no longer listen. The result is that they have developed the habit of talking past each other; they do not look at each other when they are speaking and there is very little laughter. If there is a pet dog or cat the animal is sometimes the intermediary for communication. Both are in the same room with their dog when she says, 'Fido, tell Dad that tea's ready'. These people also no longer call each other by their names, one is 'Mum' and the other is 'Dad'. If you have sunk to this level of communication you should take a good look at what has happened, but probably it is too late. Successful relationships are those in which communication is both meaningful and effective. There is no substitute for talking to each other.

Strangely, this kind of couple will stay together and one will push the other's wheelchair, but how much enjoyment has been lost? Where has the urge to continue to grow gone? The relationship no doubt is comfortable but it has no sparkle.

Get your knickers off

Old people don't have sex, do they? Of course they do and a lot of fun and pleasure can result. Get the other bits of the relationship right and there should be no problem with the sexual relationship. The older body is every bit as beautiful in its own way as the young body. Learn to enjoy its sensual pleasures. There is usually some loss of libido with advancing years so that the frequency of any sexual activity will be reduced, but the action when it happens can be great. With increasing age many men experience erectile problems and women may have a greater or lesser degree of vaginal dryness. These are perfectly normal changes but they do not mean that sexual activity cannot continue.

The nature of the sexual relationship may also change. With advancing age penetrative sex can become more difficult for the reasons already mentioned. This does not mean that orgasm cannot be achieved by one or both partners, although not necessarily on the same day. Orgasm may not always be necessary. What in the heat of youth used to be a frantic dash for the summit can become a gentle stroll through the foothills. Because you have plenty of time, and presumably nobody looking on, you can let your imaginations run free. I am not suggesting that everyone should dress in funny clothes or whatever, but you should not feel inhibited if there are things or practices that excite you. You are only old once so enjoy yourselves. And while we are on the subject, there are only two of you in the house so who needs pyjamas?

Do not be afraid of touching, because touching each other, whether publicly or in private, is the physical endorsement of an emotional bond. It is a reassurance, a way of saying, 'I care'.

Getting chemical help
There has been much advertisement of drugs to combat impotence or erectile problems in men. Such drugs, of which

Viagra is the best known, certainly work but they are not without risk. The use of Viagra, for instance, is not advised for people with heart problems. But the main problem arises from a mistaken view that to be a real man you have to have powerful erections, and it is this misunderstanding of the roles of both partners in the sexuality of older people that can lead to problems. In general, Viagra is not a remedy for a relationship that already has problems. It may also not be what is wanted. Talking with your partner openly and frankly about whatever you think is a problem in your sex life can often reveal either that there is no problem or that the problem is a different one. Before the use of any drug is considered you should discuss the whole thing and be sure that you are using the drug for the right reasons.

Family

Included in the relationships that are important are those with family, children, sometimes older parents, aunts, uncles and cousins. These relationships are so important that I have given them a whole chapter to themselves. See you on page 61.

Friends

Maintaining and enjoying friendships built up over many years is a vital component of the third age, as is the opportunity for making new friends. If you have decided to live somewhere else maintaining old friendships may become quite hard. People you saw once or twice a week you may now see only once or twice a year. You should make a serious effort to keep those long-lived friendships going because you will find that those relationships become increasingly precious as you get older. There is always the telephone or email to help sustain the links and because you have more time it may be possible to see each other more often.

True friendships survive separation and your old friends will always remain your most valued friends. You will establish new friendships in a new environment but it will be rare for them to be very close friendships, at least until several years have elapsed. You will develop a number of new acquaintances when you move somewhere else and one or two of these may eventually be called friends but it will be a slow process and not one you should try to push.

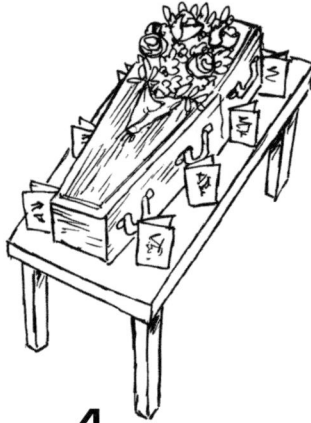

4

The difficult times

Facing loss

As you become older it becomes more and more likely you
will be faced with events or situations that are hard to endure.
One of these is bereavement; others are enforced separation
because of divorce or for health reasons. All of these involve
loss and all can and often do result in loneliness.

Bereavement

Bereavement is usually thought of as involving someone
very close to you: a partner, a child, a parent. But it may also
include the death of a more distant relative, a pet animal, a
close friend; sometimes even the death of an acquaintance.
Clearly, the death of someone very close to you will have the
greater effect but these other deaths may have a profound
effect on you also, and on your partner. You must learn how
to grieve.

In a partnership one of you will die sooner or later, leaving the other one grieving, or so you hope. The death of a partner may come at the end of a long illness and be seen as a happy release. On the other hand, death may be sudden or the result of quite a short illness and come as a shock to everyone. The first of these may be the easier to cope with and perhaps much of the grieving will already have been done during the long decline. Sudden and unexpected death may be more difficult. There may have been no opportunity for saying goodbye, and there were probably so many things yet to be done together. Family will be a help, of course; or perhaps get in the way. People will rally around — friends, and a lot of acquaintances, will call round to comfort you. This will last for about ten days! Be prepared.

Grieving

There can be no universal guide to grieving. Each of us must grieve in our own way and in our own time. But grieve we must. Some cultures are better at it than others. In some cultures the grief may be public and loud, with much wailing. Other cultures are more stolid, presenting a calm face to the world while hurting desperately inside.

My belief is that you must weep, and weep outwardly as well as inwardly. In this way you are acknowledging your grief. Do not be afraid to openly say, 'I miss him/her terribly'. Remember also that you are not alone in your grief: your children, your relatives, your friends are also grieving. Sharing your grief lifts a bit of the weight and makes the separation from your loved one more bearable.

Use the hard words

'Passed on' and 'passed away' and similar expressions are nothing phrases. Get accustomed to using the words 'dead' and 'died'. Do not try and conceal what has happened behind language that diminishes the event. Your loved one is dead; face up to it. You will find that by using the hard words the reality becomes more acceptable.

Getting through the door

Grief will stay with you for quite a long time, and it is something you will need to work at. There are a few things to understand:

▷ Ageing is inevitable and so are the losses that come with it.

▷ Life is terminal.

▷ All relationships are temporary.

▷ Grief is a door with no way around or over; you must go through it.

▷ You will live on.

▷ You can be happy again.

Getting through the door may take you up to two years and often the second year will seem the worst. Realise grief is there and do whatever you must to get through that door. Some find that closer contact with a church helps. Some busy themselves with community activities. Some write letters to themselves as a way of expressing their feelings and unloading. These are all examples of working at grief; do not be afraid of them.

Moving on

The sooner you can move on from bereavement, the sooner life can get back to normal. This does not mean that the emptiness disappears; it may last for a long time, even for ever. But there needs to be a conscious effort to return yourself to society. Put yourself in situations where you can hear laughter, see young people, smell the roses. If you belong to one or more clubs or societies put yourself in a position where you can do some committee work and include yourself in something more than your own misery. Be bold. Be positive.

Tom had cared for Marge for the last 18 months of her life as she slowly died from cancer. During this time Tom saw little of his old friends and spent much of his time doing housework, washing and cleaning as well as tending to Marge's needs. A few weeks after Marge's death a friend found Tom sitting at home looking glum. 'What's up, Tom?' asked the friend. Tom replied, 'I just don't know what to do with myself. For the last year or so I've done nothing except look after Marge.' Luckily, Tom's friends rallied around and soon had him back in society.

Not everyone has such good friends.

Children often have their own ideas about what should happen next: Mum or Dad will have to go and live near them. But this might be the wrong thing to do because, if you have a set of friends close by and several activity groups to which you belong, you should stay where you are. Perhaps you will want to move to a smaller home but stay near your pals. They may often prove to be better at getting you over the hurdle of bereavement than family.

Divorce

It is such a short word but one with a finality about it that either means relief or heartache. Divorce is never easy or quick, except in parts of the Americas. It is the public expression of the end of a relationship that may, of course, have ended some time ago. But the actual act of divorce and the subsequent *decree nisi* can be stressful and often expensive. Although a relationship may effectively have been over for months or even years for some people, the end can be a bit like bereavement. The only way to recover from the trauma of divorce is to put the whole thing behind you and move on. Easy to state, but harder to accomplish. There will be a grieving period as with any loss.

I am writing here about couples divorcing after retirement when concerns about who will have the children and so on are probably not major issues. Of course, children might have their own views about the whole thing and either take sides or accept the breakdown. Property will be split in line with the *Matrimonial Property Act* unless there is some prior contract spelling out who gets what.

Rest home for one

Another difficult time happens when one of a couple has to enter residential care, whether a rest home or a geriatric hospital. The separation can be quite similar to bereavement in its emotional effects, and the solutions also are similar. Usually the need for this separation will have been signalled well ahead of the actual event and some thought will have been given to the consequences, but not always. A sudden and unexpected severe stroke may leave little choice apart from residential care and sudden separation.

The lifestyle choices for the remaining partner are much the same as those following bereavement, the difference being that there is one of you who needs to be regularly visited and emotionally nurtured. There also may be a financial burden involved necessitating the sale of property or other assets. Such sudden events cannot be planned for in any detail but families should at least have discussed the possibility of this kind of separation and thought about their roles.

Loneliness

Loneliness is one of the biggest problems facing single older people, including those separated by forced residential care, and may often be associated with some form of depression. The whole reason for the founding of the Abbeyfield Society (see page 32) was the observation that there were a large number of lonely, single elderly sitting in their own homes with no opportunity for social interaction. The need to regularly visit a loved one in residential care can generate its own form of loneliness when there is no one else to share the load.

Loneliness is probably one of the principal reasons for the single elderly opting for a retirement village or similar. Associated with loneliness may be lack of transport and therefore limited access to those very important social occasions for social interaction, whether it be bridge, bowls, or some social club. The realisation that *being alone does not mean lonely* can be a hard one to come to but it has to happen.

The one thing that must not be permitted is sitting at home wallowing in self-pity and undergoing slow, or even rapid, decay. It is up to family, friends and whatever support groups exist within the community to ensure that this worst of states does not occur. Always there is someone who knows that a single older person is isolated and probably very lonely. Very often that someone is another older person.

Marrying again

One solution for loneliness used by some single elderly is remarriage. This may not be the stated reason, but loneliness frequently is the real reason for remarriage. Be very careful because this step may result in more heartache than it resolves. If you live in a small community you may not be forgiven, and I have been told of instances where this has occurred, with the result that the new couple have had to move elsewhere.

Bill's wife died and Alice's husband had died a year before. They lived in the same small town and both were very popular in the community. Six months after Bill's wife died they decided to get married. Because they were known and liked, the community accepted this arrangement and everyone was delighted.

Small towns can be funny places. Had Alice and Bill lived in a city they might not have had to satisfy the community that what they wanted to do was acceptable.

Then there is the question of property. Usually on remarriage there are two sets of offspring to be considered, both with some expectations of inheritance; an expectation that should not be denied. Any couple considering remarriage, or even moving in together in some sort of partnership, should get separate legal advice and, if necessary, have a contract drawn up that clearly states the property rights and who gets what in the case of death or separation.

Losing the car

One thing you do have to plan for is the day when you are no longer able to drive. If you live any distance from shops or public transport, you will face major difficulties if you cannot use your own car. Of course, if your husband or wife can still drive there is less of a problem. But what if your partner cannot drive either? There are some people who, for whatever reason, have never learnt or choose not to drive. If one of these is your partner there is a clear problem. Losing the right to drive will happen to many people and you may be one of them, but by preparing well ahead you may be able to soften the blow.

An obvious step is to move so that you live somewhere close to public transport, and this is one of the things to consider when it comes to choosing where to live. Many retirement complexes have transport available, usually a minibus or similar. But this might not always be there when you want it. You should not put yourself at the mercy of friends or relatives. Find your own solution and do it before the terrible day comes when you can no longer drive a car.

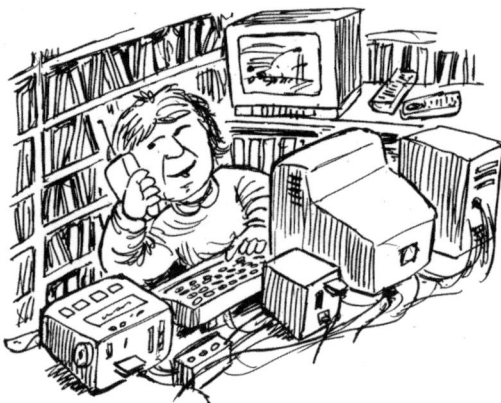

5

All by yourself

Living alone

It is quite likely that you will be forced to live alone for some part of your old age. This is more so for women than for men because, on the whole, women live longer than men. Nevertheless, some men will have to face the prospect of living by themselves. For everyone, living alone after years of being in a partnership is a major challenge that can only be met head on and positively.

*Being alone does not and
must not mean lonely.*

There is a very real risk that people living by themselves become socially isolated. This must not be allowed to happen to you. You need to behave as though nothing has changed:

▷ Follow your old social routines.

▷ Keep in close touch with your friends.

▷ Go regularly to the meetings of your clubs/societies.

▷ Do not move away from your established friends
   unless there are compelling reasons.

There probably will be some pressure from your family to move closer to them. This may be a good thing but only if you can maintain your friendships. Provided you are reasonably healthy you will be better off staying where you are. But this might still mean that you should change your living arrangements. Unless you are totally passionate about gardening there are good reasons for moving from your villa into a more secure environment— an apartment or a townhouse. You might want to consider a retirement complex if there is a suitable one in your area, or possibly an Abbeyfield house.

If you do decide to change your residence you should make the effort to furnish your new place in a way that suits you rather than just moving some or all of the furniture from your former home. There may be some things that you are not prepared to part with; things that are either precious to you or you need. Minimise them. Take only what you absolutely must have and sell or give away the rest. The idea is that you are going to start again; the place you will move into is yours and no one else's.

One house is better than two

House sharing can be a good way for old friends to both economise and combat loneliness. Why rattle around separately in two houses when combining assets, and sometimes skills, in one house can make life a lot easier? The friends can be same sex or different; the principles are the same. In this instance no romance is involved or intended; the arrangement is for mutual benefit and nothing else. However, there still may remain some legal issues and it is important for both parties to seek legal advice before setting up such an arrangement.

Here is another solution:

Bob and his wife and Sally and her husband had lived next door to each other for years and the two couples had become very close friends. Sadly, one husband and one wife died leaving Bob and Sally alone and a bit lonely. Rather than move into one house they decided to stay as they were but go to social things, the theatre, and out with other friends together when they felt like it. They even went travelling together. There was no suggestion of romance or marriage and both were very happy with their arrangement.

Get skills

Living alone entails doing as many things as possible yourself. For many people this should not be a problem because they may well have been doing everything themselves during the terminal illness of a partner. The really prepared people will have made a point of learning how to manage the home and the financial affairs before things go wrong.

Women need to know:

  ▷ bank details

  ▷ investment details

  ▷ how to pay accounts

  ▷ how to change a light bulb

▷ how to programme a video recorder or work the DVD player

▷ how to work the computer.

Men need to know:

▷ how to cook tasty and healthy meals

▷ how to iron

▷ how to work the washing machine and dishwasher

▷ all the same things as women.

In an ideal partnership both should know how to do all these things and share the doing of them. But often the traditional lines are drawn and any former skills are lost. Try hard to match the ideal.

Animal friends

Pets can be very rewarding for those living by themselves. Most people will choose either a cat or a dog but some might quite like a cage bird. Whichever of these you decide on, or even all, take care in your choice of breed, bearing in mind your ability to cope with a vigorous, demanding mastiff, the nocturnal wanderings of the typical alley cat or the constant, 'Who's a pretty boy?' of a parrot.

Pets are:

▷ company

▷ aids to movement

▷ sources of humour

▷ possible security devices, if they bark.

Pets need:

▷ training

▷ food

▷ water

▷ exercise

▷ grooming

▷ somewhere to sleep other than your bed

▷ health care.

The importance of training, particularly for dogs, cannot be stressed enough. There is nothing worse than a badly trained, or even untrained, dog. If you do get a dog it is a good idea to go to puppy socialisation sessions where the youngster can become used to the company of other dogs. Then you can proceed to local dog-training classes. These are not expensive but are of great benefit. You will find that it is probably you rather than the dog who ends up being trained! Your local veterinary service will know how to get into these classes.

Pets are a responsibility and when you are away from the house or apartment there will have to be somewhere for them to shelter and have water. Cats are easier at this than dogs and can usually be left all day happily fending for themselves. Dogs need more care, should not be left for long periods of time, and are not very suitable for an apartment. If you go away often you probably should not have a pet. Continually being put into a boarding kennel or cattery does not make for good pet-human relationships.

Keep fit

This comes up under other headings but it is particularly important for those living alone because of their tendency to become isolated. There is no substitute for walking in the fresh air even if you are walking to the gym, stopping occasionally during your walk to swipe at a golf ball, being active on the bowling or croquet green, or going off to do some shopping. Not doing these things means that you really are becoming socially isolated and also likely to become less healthy.

Things spiritual

A number of people who live alone find that a return to the church, or the discovery of the church, is of great benefit. If you already are a member of some community of faith you may want to play a more active part in that community and take advantage of the networks of support that exist within it. If you have no such links you may have a friend or a relative who is involved in some church and who can introduce you. In most communities there are several active religious groups that are always ready to provide support through a variety of means such as regular meetings, social outings, informal gatherings, and so on. Do not neglect this potentially rewarding part of your life.

Live well

It is important for those living alone, as well as everyone else, that standards are maintained. Dress well, not necessarily expensively but well. Take pride in your appearance, spoil yourself and wear a bit of colour. Above all, do not let yourself become scruffy. If you believe that the outside world thinks you look good you will also feel good. The same applies to your living surroundings. Keep the place clean and acceptably tidy. Do the washing regularly as well as the ironing. Feed yourself properly and give yourself a treat from time to time. There is more to life than baked beans and sausages; shun takeaways like the plague. Eat well, and drink well too if you wish. Entertain friends to dinner, lunch, or a barbecue. By following these positive things you will be able to take pleasure in living alone.

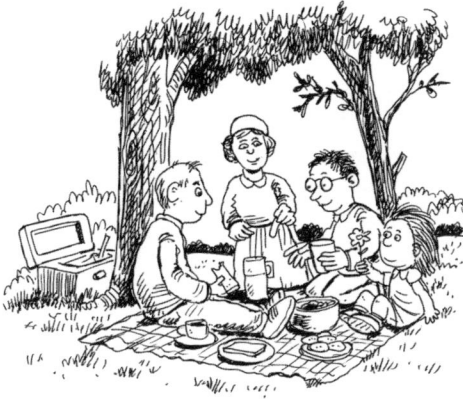

6

Caught in the middle

Families

It is no longer unusual for there to be two generations in retirement. Naturally those now retiring feel a responsibility for their older parents, any number between one and four, but they will also feel some responsibility to the two younger generations growing behind them. In this way the retiring couple is caught in the middle with responsibilities, or at least allegiances, in every direction. When you add in aunts and uncles, cousins, nieces and nephews, not to mention great-aunts and great-uncles, the kinship total starts to get very large.

But even if you are the only generation in retirement the third age has the potential to bring with it stronger and more extended family ties. Children and grandchildren form the close family that you are likely to spend the most time with but you may find yourself seeing more of cousins, and aunts and uncles if they are still around. Being retired provides the opportunity to have grandchildren to stay and to enjoy the rewards that having young people around you bring. Grandparents and grandchildren often bond very closely and get a lot of pleasure from each other. A comedian once remarked that this is because they share a common enemy! Take care though that you do not become a convenient dumping place.

The extended family as network

For the great majority of people, gone are the days when there could be three generations living under one roof. For many of us the extended family living together, or in close proximity, is a thing of the past even though there may be a definable extended family that has some form of communication within itself. This extended family can form a network of support for those who become ill or suffer loss.

Family can provide:

▷ friendship

▷ compassion

▷ love

▷ support in the home or garden

▷ assistance with transport

▷ a resource for family history.

As more and more family members live into old age this support network starts to become increasingly important, so everyone needs to try to ensure the communication lines remain open and functioning. The network can be a powerful influence both for those who are old and for the younger generations. Develop it and use it.

Problems happen

Although the third age is a time when many families come closer together, it can also be a time of stress when those in the younger generation get into trouble, usually with their own relationships or financially. These problems can be worrying for the older generation who feel that somehow they should be helping. Probably it is best not to become too closely involved but there are no rules. Every situation will be different demanding different solutions. But the older generation is usually the stable rock that provides reassurance.

Not everyone within a family necessarily gets on with everyone else. Sometimes tensions develop and have to be faced, or walked away from. There may be arguments about inheritances — *'Where there's a will there's a family'* — or other family squabbles. Stay out of them if you can. Deal with them if you cannot.

Grandparents as parents

It happens. Sometimes the only solution to a problem that has struck the children is for the grandparents to look after the grandchildren. This should not be permitted to become a long-term arrangement because it is doubtful whether it is in the best interests of either the grandchildren or the grandparents, especially as everyone grows older. Try for a quick and satisfactory solution.

The generation above you

You may well have one or several ageing parents. These older folk can be a source of pleasure and also a source of concern as they become ill or simply frail. Often they will be facing decisions about their care: questions about retirement complexes or rest homes will arise and you probably will be expected to contribute to the debate. Support for them can take up quite a lot of your time and you need to be sure that they are receiving all their entitlements for care. Do not let your own life or lives be swamped by caring for these elderly people, especially if there are no other siblings who can share the burden. It is far better that professional carers do the job if it means you can get your life back.

Decorating the family tree

Many people in the third age start to take an interest in their family histories and start on the genealogy trail. This can be both time-consuming and rewarding. There are now many websites that help you trace family trees, and most public libraries have documents that can be useful for tracing particular individuals. Once individuals are identified birth certificates can be obtained, for a small fee, from the Department of Internal Affairs. There are several quite powerful computer programs to aid you in constructing a family tree, and many communities have genealogical clubs or societies with members who know all about the software. By joining one of these you can rapidly learn how to go about tracing your own family. Aunts and uncles are a useful source of information and often know details of the family that your parents may not have known or perhaps had not thought important enough to pass on.

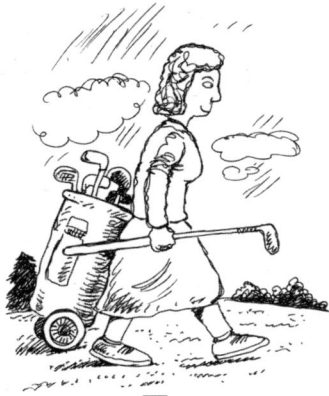

7

Filling the day

Staying active

People are not statues built to stand still and do nothing. We all have some compulsion to do things even if these are trivial and of no practical use to anyone, not even ourselves. But there are many people who are motivated to keeping themselves busy in some way or another that does result in use to somebody. Retirement from their profession or trade brings with it the need to replace the 40-hour working week with some equivalent, or lesser, time devoted to one or more activities that may or may not earn money. Very few, if any, successfully retired people have not replaced one occupation with another. It may not be full-time, it may not even bring in extra income, but it will be a task, or series of tasks, that fill most of the day and bring satisfaction.

It is no good waking up on that fateful Monday morning and asking yourself, or your partner, what you are going to do. You should know in advance what sort of thing you want to do and, most importantly, who the people are that can help you achieve it. This doesn't mean you should be leaping out of bed on that Monday morning and dashing off to get stuck into some worthwhile task. This means you should have a broad idea of the kinds of things you might do and how to go about doing them. In other words, you have planned and prepared yourself.

Letting go

However good the preparation, whatever the new activities are going to be, many people on stopping the work they have been doing for years find it difficult to let go. For some it is a little like bereavement and these people genuinely grieve. There are no magic remedies. But those who have planned and those who do have alternative activities will find it easier to let go than those who have not done these things. Letting go can take quite a long time; it is a little like giving up a habit such as smoking. In time the craving wears off and you can stop feeling guilty about not being at your desk or wherever. Although you may have made many friends among your workmates, or at least think you have, do not expect them to call round to see how you are getting on. Only your true friends will do that. Once you have left the workplace you will largely be forgotten. Get used to it. It might hurt a bit to start with but you'll get over it. It is another part of letting go.

Plan to be active

Everyone should aim to have some kind of activity, paid or unpaid. It may not always be possible to plan this in any detail, unless you happen to continue living in the same place. But, if you are going to move to another community, it will not always be possible to immediately find the kind of thing you'd like to do. Try and think creatively and do not choose exactly the same line of work you were in before retirement. However, the skills you have developed over the years should not be wasted; just steer them in a different direction. Don't be afraid to accept a lower paid or less responsible job. Even part-time is better than no time at all; and what about job sharing? Some employers may be glad to take on your skills but not want the hassle of a new full-time employee. Here the possibilities are probably great but mostly unexplored. Presumably a different employer is going to want to use at least some of the skills you have gained. Skills obtained in one industry can often be put to use in a completely different trade.

Paid work is not the only activity available. If you do not need to supplement your income, you might choose to spend your time doing other things, or even a mix of things.

Here are a few possible activities:

▷ income-producing work

▷ intellectual pursuits

▷ community service activities and clubs

▷ sports and recreation — get physical

▷ religious activities

▷ crafts — be creative

▷ hobbies

▷ travel — roam the world.

Income-producing work

Sometimes what was previously a five-day-a-week job can become a part-time job with hours to suit yourself. This can be a very good solution both for those who can manage it and for their employers. Some income is retained, skills are put to good use, interest is maintained and time is freed up for other things. In this way, if you are fortunate you may be able to slowly ease yourself into retirement by remaining in your job, or a related job, within the company you work for but working reduced hours, perhaps job sharing, over an agreed period of a few months or years. Some employers are starting to realise the benefits this kind of arrangement can have for the company; there can be many advantages in having someone around with long experience and good skills. *Old is not useless.*

Other employers have not yet woken up to these advantages but it is likely that more will as skilled labour shortages start to bite. If your employer does not have such a scheme available, you should try talking to your boss some months before you plan to retire, or the company pushes you out, to find out if a reduced working arrangement would be possible. With a little creative thought and some flexibility a satisfactory agreement usually can be reached.

A different job

Even if you leave your former job you do not have to completely stop doing what you are, or were, good at. Part-time work may be attractive for many reasons. On the other hand, you may not want to continue in your previous line of work and may want to do something completely different — like the bank manager wanting to be a motor mechanic. If that is your thing, go for it if the opportunity presents. But you will not achieve your dream without planning ahead.

You will need to set up the opportunities, perhaps even do some preliminary training in your spare time. You will fail if you think you can buy a plot of land, plant 300 olive trees and then find out how to grow, prune the trees, harvest and process your fruit. Do the research first. Find out if what you want to do will really work. Maybe olives are not the best crop on that particular plot. Maybe you should think about planting a different variety. Be prepared to admit your mistakes and modify your plans.

You may even decide you would like to run your own small business, buy a franchise or a bookshop and fill the day behind a counter. Good for you, but be sure you can afford to have some free time as well.

Bob and Carol bought a shoe shop in a good location in a good suburb. Bob previously had worked a 40-hour week while Carol had worked part-time. For the first year or two things went very well; the shop made money and they both enjoyed working. In fact, things went so well that they opened a second shop in another suburb. Soon both of them were working far more than 40-hour weeks and becoming quite stressed, sometimes with each other. Eventually, they decided they could afford to put managers in both shops and take some time out for themselves. They are still enjoying the income, working 20-hour weeks and starting to live, and love, again. Bob thinks they should have thought ahead a bit more and put at least one manager in when they opened the second shop. The financial return would have been less and so would have the stress.

Intellectual pursuits

Under this heading there are several choices:

▷ exploring the computer

▷ attending further education courses

▷ taking up writing

▷ going to the library.

This list is not exhaustive. Some people might include improving skill at chess or bridge, doing jigsaw puzzles, collecting books or antiques.

Exploring the computer

The computer has become a part of everyday life for many people. For older people a computer, usually a PC, with an Internet connection can be a great way to keep in touch with family and friends. For retired people without computer skills there is an organisation called Seniornet. Seniornet provides classes in computer use for older people taught by other older people; people who have themselves been through the process. Most areas in the country have a Seniornet group and many University of the Third Age groups (see page 124) have computer classes that may provide much the same sort of thing. There really is nothing worse than acquiring a device that you cannot get the best out of, and the modern computer has a wealth of things to offer.

However, while it can be very helpful to have someone show you the basics of using a computer, finding out the possibilities yourself can be the really rewarding thing as well as putting your mind to work. Remember, *old does not mean dumb*. The Consumers' Institute has available a good little book called *easypcprojects* and it is well worth investing in this or something similar so that you have a reference close to hand. Such books can set you on the road to further exploring the potentials of your machine.

Get caught in the web

It is interesting that family and friends communicating by email often write much longer letters than they would if writing by hand. This is one of the good things about email and the Internet. Not only can you spread yourself at low cost, but your communication is virtually instantaneous, leaving aside the differences in time zones. The Internet also opens up a whole world of information. Sure, sometimes it can all get a bit frustrating but what you want to know will be there somewhere.

There are several search engines; that is, sites that allow you to search for particular subjects. They include Google, Yahoo and Altavista. The addresses of these and a few others along with some interesting websites are listed on page 125. The search engines take a bit of getting used to and you may end up with a whole lot of stuff that you do not need or want, but by refining your searches you can get just what you are looking for. Of the engines listed Google is probably the most frequently used and it is very powerful. Some people seem to spend almost the whole day googling!

Apart from the various search engines it is useful to have the web addresses of a number of key sites that can provide a lot of useful information. Increasingly, people are using the Internet to make travel arrangements. You can now book airline tickets, hotel and motel rooms, bus tours and much else worldwide. As with googling, it is possible to spend hours just browsing the sites and planning where to go next. There are also a number of locally produced Internet guide magazines and general computer magazines available that contain a lot of useful information as well as a lot of gobbledegook!

Don't become a recluse

While a computer — whether the cheaper PC (bulky) or notebook or laptop — can be of considerable use, it can also become a fairly anti-social device. This is particularly true if the computer is kept in the third or fourth bedroom away from the mainstream of the house. The best place by far for the machine is in the living area so that the person using it is not out of contact with the rest of the family. Another problem with computers is the temptation to waste time in a monumental way. Games can be addictive as well as enjoyable. 'Hold on, dear. I'll just have one more try,' usually leads to at least three, or ten, more tries!

Go digital

If you have a digital camera a computer is almost a necessity as you can download images, edit them and send them all over the world. The technology is amazing and exciting, and you should take full advantage of these devices.

Attending further education courses

One of the benefits of the third age is that there is time to learn something new. Many people reach retirement wishing they had learned more about this or that in school, or they had had the time to follow up something that always had interested them. Now you *do* have the time and now you *can* do something about learning whatever it is that interests you. The possibilities are huge. Here are some ideas:

▷ tertiary courses

▷ secondary school evening classes

▷ specialist clubs and societies

▷ University of the Third Age.

Tertiary courses
Universities and technical institutes offer a large variety of learning opportunities. Although one or two of you could be interested in completing a degree in astrophysics, the rest do not have to go that far. All of these institutions allow you to take selected papers, often on a part-time basis or even extramurally. The possibilities are too numerous to list here but a good starting place is the list of selected institutions in Want more? (see page 124).

Secondary school evening classes
Many secondary schools run evening classes on a variety of topics, sometimes craft-related. These are usually advertised by mail drop or in your local, community newspaper. Mostly these classes offer short duration courses with no qualifications at the end, and people take them in order to improve certain skills or simply out of interest. If the local high school or college does offer these classes, it is worth keeping an eye out for something that might be interesting.

Specialist clubs and societies
Wherever you live there are likely to be many clubs or societies devoted to a particular area of interest. There are bridge clubs, chess clubs, gardening clubs, numismatic societies, philatelic societies and various hobby clubs. These clubs welcome new members and particularly those who have little or no knowledge of the topic. Such clubs can be an invaluable source of new activities and also a source of new friends. Don't be afraid; join them.

University of the Third Age

This movement started many years ago in France and has spread worldwide, changing a bit in the process. University of the Third Age (U3A) is widely represented in New Zealand with about 50 groups. U3A provides learning opportunities for older people without the need for pre-requisites and providing no qualifications at the end; there is a significant social component to the meetings. U3A groups may include local history, creative writing, geology, genealogy, language learning, art appreciation and so on. For the most part, all learning-group meetings are held in someone's home and during daylight hours. *U3Aonline*, based in Australia, also offers various courses available on the Internet at a small cost for those who live in remote areas. This is accessible from New Zealand.

Taking up writing

Almost everyone has at some time read a book or a magazine article and thought, 'I'm sure I could have written that better'. Now you have the chance to do just that. Writing can be purely for pleasure, it can be because you have something to say and want others to know your opinion, or because you have technical knowledge that you want to share.

There are several things you might try:

▷ letters to the newspaper

▷ magazine articles

▷ poetry

▷ short stories

▷ a novel

▷ the story of your life

▷ the story of somebody else's life

▷ the history of your town or family

▷ a book like this.

Whatever you choose you must develop a discipline so that you write something every day. Try to set aside a particular time in the day devoted to writing and stick to it rigidly. It may be that most of that time is spent looking out the window; no matter, as long as you get those few words on to paper. To help develop your writing skills there may be evening classes available in your locality. U3As usually have a creative writing group where others like you are grappling with the muse.

Going to the library
This a good place to introduce you to your local library. The library offers the opportunity to seriously widen your reading horizons, an opportunity that many in the third age take. Even if your local library is quite small you can order books from a much larger resource, the national library service. Your library usually has a computerised catalogue enabling you to search for the titles you might want or even through subjects to find what titles exist.

Of course, you will not want to spend your whole time reading, but an hour or two a day with your nose in a good book can be a very pleasurable experience. Some may find all their pleasure in fiction; others delve into history or biography. Your library has something for everyone. And there are not just books. Most libraries now have a stock of CDs available for borrowing so you can even listen as you read!

Community service activities and clubs

Within every community there are many volunteer tasks that need to be done. Very frequently these are done by the retired. They include:

▷ staffing the local library

▷ driving for Age Concern

▷ delivering meals on wheels

▷ staffing citizens advice bureaus

▷ taking administration roles in clubs and societies.

The list can be a long one. Every community has a range of activities in which you can join. For some there will be golf, tennis, croquet, walking, fishing, and much, much more. More sedentary are bridge, other card games, chess, mahjong and so on. Likewise, every community has clubs and societies, sometimes associated with these pastimes, sometimes more general. There are:

▷ church groups

▷ Probus clubs

▷ Grey Power

▷ Age Concern

▷ 60s Up movement

▷ senior citizens clubs

▷ gardening clubs

▷ sports clubs

▷ games clubs

▷ travel clubs.

Some of these will be considered in more detail, and as you can see quite a few are devoted to older people. No one need ever feel isolated within our communities with all these opportunities at hand. And yet a surprising number of people seem to find it very difficult to take the first step in joining a club or society, especially when they have moved to a new community. Reading this will not allow you to overcome your fear of the unknown but, if you have read this far, perhaps you will have developed a positive attitude and go out and do it.

Become a Probian

There are about 50,000 members of Probus Clubs in New Zealand. Probus, which stands for professional and business, is a social club that meets monthly, usually with one or more speakers, and provides a great opportunity to meet people of your own age, people with a wide variety of backgrounds and interests. Many Probus clubs also have interest groups such as walking, singing or games.

Probus clubs are sometimes called geriatric Rotary and it is true that Rotary clubs are instrumental in the initial formation of Probus clubs. However, the members of Probus clubs are not drawn exclusively from the ranks of Rotary and they include people from all walks of life; anyone who wishes to join is welcome, although you need to be proposed.

The power of grey

Grey Power is mainly an advocacy group for the welfare and rights of older people, but membership also offers a number of discounts for various services. Grey Power groups meet regularly and provide social opportunities as well as advocacy.

Age Concern has less of an advocacy role, and is less of

a social group, but is still concerned with the health and well-being of older people. Some Age Concern councils also run a number of activities for older people such as driving courses, social occasions, falls prevention courses and other activities aimed at helping older people live a good life.

The 60s Up movement and senior citizens clubs are not represented in every locality but there is often one or other of them wherever you are. Mostly these organisations offer social contact, indoor games, speakers and outings. Some have walking groups.

Membership of all these organisations is not costly, and to belong to one or more can be very stimulating and provide a way to meet new people. With all of these groups, clubs and societies there is always the opportunity to help out in some way. Most change their officers every year and members can get the most out of their club by helping to administer the club's affairs. Don't be afraid — stand for office.

Once you know the opportunities that exist in your community perhaps you will be stimulated to take the plunge. There are some very nice and caring people out there; people who will be as interested in meeting you as you will be in meeting them. You will soon make new friends and gradually grow into the community. It is probably true that being accepted into most small communities can be difficult. Sometimes it may take several years. Joining things is a way of speeding up the process.

Get physical

Exercise, exercise and more exercise are among the key ingredients of a long and healthy life. Most able-bodied people enjoy some sort of sport, competitive or not. The third age is an ideal time to spend practising, playing or indulging in your favourite sport or sports, or doing something to keep yourself fit. The opportunities are too great to list but things like bowls (lawn, indoor or ten-pin), golf, sailing or boating, fishing (salt or fresh water), croquet and tennis are all things that older people can enjoy if fit enough. Such activities have the added advantage of maintaining fitness. Many community groups include a walking group and, as walking is great exercise, these groups are well worth joining. Not only do you get the exercise, but also you get it in good company. Another possibility is to join a gym. Some offer aerobics for older people as well as tailored fitness programmes.

Some light recreation

As well as sports there are other recreational activities available in most communities. These include bridge and other card games, mahjong and chess, snooker at the club among others. There are clubs devoted to these recreations and all are happy to provide instruction to beginners.

Sports clubs and recreational clubs share with the community clubs and societies a need for administration and there is an opportunity, sometimes an obligation, to become involved in this.

Religious activities

As well as regular devotional services, many churches have educational or social groups rather similar to the community groups listed above. In addition, there are opportunities to assist in the management of church affairs and to help with keeping the church and church hall clean and tidy. Some religious communities have regular retreats or other activities for those who wish for more than the weekly service.

Become creative

What would you like to spend time doing?

- ▷ oil painting
- ▷ watercolour painting
- ▷ pottery
- ▷ ceramic painting
- ▷ sculpture
- ▷ weaving
- ▷ tapestry
- ▷ quilting
- ▷ cabinetmaking
- ▷ metalwork.

It is all there if you want it, even bookbinding and leather work. Plenty of people and classes are available to help you get started or brush up your skills. Most communities have groups devoted to at least some of the above creative crafts. So, if you are feeling the urge to create, or just dabble, take the plunge.

Hobbies

We all were encouraged to have them when we were children and some of us continued them throughout our lives. I wonder how many half-filled stamp albums lurk in dusty cupboards or were thrown away when shifting house? Hobbies come in all shapes and sizes: from restoring traction engines to hunting native orchids with almost everything in between. When they enter the third age some people, the real enthusiasts, breathe a sigh of relief and settle down to convert their part-time hobby into a full-time occupation. But most people will either start up a new hobby, perhaps collecting of some kind, or resurrect a hobby they once quite enjoyed. The latter will not want to spend all day doing whatever the hobby requires, but will be perfectly happy spending an hour or two when the opportunity presents pottering with their coin collection or whatever.

This is not to belittle the place of hobbies; they are a good way to exercise both body and minds and there is much enjoyment to be had. Most hobbies are catered for through societies or clubs, many of which have websites. So, dig out the stamp album and the collection of health stamp first-day covers and start up again.

Roam the world

Visiting places you previously have never been to can be one of the great joys of retirement. The world trip, the extended luxury cruise, an adventure holiday if the body is up to it (and most are) can all be worthwhile. Even travelling closer to home can have its pleasures, and often the best places to visit can be found quite close to home.

Travel abroad will be on most people's list for retirement, and a good thing it is too. There are all kinds of packages for tours of here, there and everywhere. Often a package tour of a country or region enables you to decide which places you would wish to concentrate on in a later visit. A tour of Europe, for example, may make you want to spend at least a week in Rome, or two weeks in Moscow, Prague or Paris.

There are also 'theme tours' that focus on such things as regional cuisine, wine, art, music, architecture and history. These are becoming more common and provide educational opportunities as well as travel. Very often these tours stimlate tours or individual trips to other places.

The Internet is invaluable when it comes to travel. Airlines and tour companies have websites, and often booking your travel, your tour and your accommodation can be done on the Internet. Travel agents, of course, offer a personal and tailored service but the more adventurous should certainly spend some time searching the web for opportunities and bargains.

Be sure to insure

Travel to other countries has its hazards, and insurance, particularly health, is essential. The cost can be quite high and rises as you get older. If you do not have health insurance the costs of private medical treatment can be astronomical in many countries, particularly the United States. If you do not use the private service in many countries you will not get very good treatment, but note that reciprocal public hospital services exist for Australia and the United Kingdom.

Several gold credit cards offer a complimentary travel insurance package, usually with an excess of about $200, which still may be less than with other policies. You must always declare existing medical conditions, even if you believe they do not present a problem. The penalties for ignoring this are dire and may cost you many thousands of dollars. The advice from the Consumers' Institute is to shop around and give yourself plenty of time to do so.

All this gloom aside it is possible to have many enjoyable travel experiences. Be bold — don't always go for the obvious: try the Trans-Siberian railway; go to Europe or the United States in the owner's cabin on a cargo ship; take one or more of the great Australian train journeys; visit China, India, South America, Namibia — the possibilities are, well, as big as the world really. It all just needs a bit of research, thought and planning.

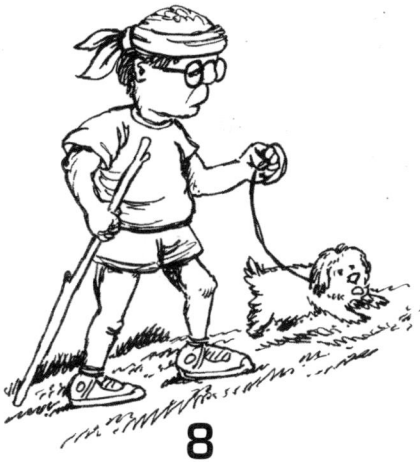

8

Looking after the body

Keeping healthy

It is a regrettable fact that as we age we begin to suffer small, or even large, component failure. Eyesight dims, hearing fades, joints become painful, hearts stop working properly and so on. Health now and in the future is an important part of preparing for retirement. You may be able to play tennis and golf or ski now, but will this still be so in five years time? Your health status has a bearing on where to live, what activities you can involve yourself in, and what you must avoid.

It makes little sense, after suffering a serious illness that is likely to recur, going to live a long way away from a major hospital and buying a property with a steep garden needing a lot of hard work. But there are people who have done just that. At the same time, a setback in health should not be a reason to panic, sell up and go to live next to a hospital.

Health, or lack of it, should not be the sole reason for making a decision unless it is life threatening. Be sensible, talk to your health professionals, whether in general practice or specialising, and respect their advice even if for some reason you choose not to take it. Just make sure that the 'some reason' is a very compelling one.

The choices you have when faced with deteriorating health are many and very often depend on what is wrong with you. There may have to be some modification of the home; for instance, if you or your partner are in a wheelchair. As you and your partner become older and creakier it probably becomes more important to think of downsizing your property. Will you still need four bedrooms when you are 85? Will you be able to keep up the garden when you are 80? Is it retirement village time? But all this doesn't mean you are on the scrap heap. You can still have a satisfying life even though some bits of you may be failing. Again, as it is in the third age, it is all a matter of attitude, if you think you are ready for the scrap heap you probably are and you will not last much longer. Believe that you still have a lot of good years left in you and you probably will live to enjoy them.

Get ahead of health while you can

There are a number of potentially expensive health-related matters that you should attend to before you retire. Eyesight is all important. If you think you are going to need new glasses, or even your first pair, the time to get them is while you have the money. The same goes for a hearing aid. Dental treatment is not covered by many health insurers so make sure you get your teeth and general oral hygiene in as good a state as possible, and any crowns done before you actually stop earning.

Joint replacements are expensive things, and many of us

need them if we are going to stay capable of active living. Again, if your joints, particularly shoulders, hips and knees are beginning to cause you pain and disability, it would be wise to have the appropriate X-rays, consult an orthopaedic surgeon and even perhaps have an MRI scan. If it turns out that you could benefit from a joint replacement, do not be tempted to put the day off. Go ahead and get it done.

There are other health problems that also may benefit from early action: varicose veins, hernias and so on. The whole objective of all this is to ensure that you start your retirement in the best possible physical shape, and that you are therefore unlikely to face expensive treatment bills, at least in the short to medium term.

Whatever your health status you must try to keep yourself physically and mentally as fit as possible. This does not necessarily mean lots of full-on exercise, going to the gym, although you may decide you would like to do that. It does mean remaining active by:

▷ walking rather than riding whenever you can

▷ keeping the remote next to the television

▷ parking the car some way from the shops so you have to walk

▷ playing some active sport

▷ keeping the mind going.

In many communities there are walking groups, either independent or associated with some group such as Probus or the 60s Up movement. These are good to join because you will be exercising with others of your own age, or older, and the experience of walking along new tracks can be very satisfying. Walking really is a 'best exercise' especially as you grow older so buy a pair of suitable walking shoes and stride out.

Give up puffing

Stopping smoking is obvious but very difficult — get whatever help you can. The various nicotine substitute products can be helpful but at the end of the day it is only your own desire to quit that will enable you to succeed. There are courses available for those who really want to stop but are finding it hard. Acupuncture or hypnosis can be of help for some people.

Look after the teeth

Eat sensibly and keep your teeth in good condition. You cannot eat properly if you cannot chew. Just because you have moved away doesn't mean you have to drive 200 kilometres to your old dentist. There really are very good dentists in small towns. However, dentistry is not cheap so a regular visit to a dental hygienist is well worth the trouble and the lesser expense. Many dentists now have a hygienist associated with their practice.

Keep the senses in order
I can't read the instructions

Eyes and ears also need attention. Reading is a pleasure and should not be made difficult. As we get older we need more light to read by and we need to be able to read comfortably in that light. Make sure you are using the correct spectacles. Although the relatively cheap reading glasses that can be bought at many retail outlets are very good, they may not correct all your vision faults. A check by an optometrist from time to time will exclude glaucoma and cataract as concerns, and also make sure that you are using the spectacles that are right for you. The optometrist will tell you if the cheaper reading glasses are suitable or if you need better lenses for comfortable reading or for long distance vision. One of the greatest fears older people have is that they might lose their driving licence because of failing eyesight. By going for regular checks serious loss of vision, such as with the condition of macular degeneration, can often be averted or successfully treated.

What was that you said?

Hearing likewise deteriorates with age: noisy rooms are avoided because you cannot hear what the person speaking to you is saying; music becomes more difficult to listen to. Seek advice and do not be afraid to admit that things are not quite what they were. Maybe you will need a hearing aid. Maybe it is something else. An audiologist would be a good place to start. The audiologist will examine your ears and test your hearing. There may be an accumulation of wax plugging the ear canal and muffling sound, a condition often fixed by using a wax softener from the pharmacy. If you have anything more serious, the audiologist will advise you to seek specialist advice. Don't put off attending to things to do with health. If you have a problem, get it seen to. Consult the professionals.

Get under cover

Health insurance can be of great benefit as age increases. Many of the annoying things that go wrong — eyesight, hearing, joints, varicose veins and hernias — are not easily or speedily treated within the free health service. Yet it is these supposedly minor problems that can be a significant cause of discomfort and disability for older people. With appropriate health insurance treatment is quick, effective, and not costly; except for the premiums. Here there is a clear choice: spend the money on health insurance and be comfortable knowing you can get the best treatment without waiting, or salt the cash away and endure discomfort and disability in the hope that one day it can be fixed. Don't forget that by the time your disability is really severe your general health may also have deteriorated, making recovery that much more difficult. If you can afford it, get health insurance. Unfortunately, not everyone will be able to afford private cover. For those who can't there can be little comfort in knowing that they will get good treatment within the public system if they are seriously ill, when the small things that make life uncomfortable have to be left untreated.

Most health insurers offer several levels of cover and most increase their premiums with increasing age. In addition, most will not cover you for pre-existing conditions, although some may waive this if you do not claim for that condition, and have had no further problems for a number of years. The cover offered is usually either comprehensive, meaning you are covered for all or most health expenses, or 'hospital only', which covers specialist fees and hospital expenses. Once you have passed the age of 60 the advice is to have hospital-only cover and pay for visits to your family doctor and for prescriptions yourself as such costs are relatively small. You also might wish to consider a plan that carries some excess — you pay the first $500, for example. With such plans the premiums will be lower but the major expenses will still be covered.

Useful information
A couple of websites are helpful sources of information about health services for the elderly. The Eldernet site, mentioned

previously, has information on many other things concerned with the health and well-being of the elderly, while Weka has a lot of information about services, mainly for those with a disability but relevant for many others as well.

Thinking straight

Keeping the mind going is an essential ingredient of a healthy life. The phrase 'use it or lose it' appears to apply just as much to the mind as it does to the body. Crossword puzzles, computer games, card and board games all help to keep your mind active and your memory in good shape. Make sure that you do not overtax your brain; as an organ it uses quite a lot of blood and a surprising amount of energy. If you find yourself making a few mistakes at some task, take a break, and give the brain a rest. Do some stretching exercises, particularly for the upper part of the body and you will find that your concentration improves as a result.

I can't remember

It is a common belief that memory declines with age, and to some extent this is true. But the kinds of things that are remembered also change with age. Older people have a wealth of knowledge stemming from their experiences over the years and they tend to retain this knowledge. They may not remember the dates of important battles, or a complete list of New Zealand prime ministers (who does?), but they are able to transmit their knowledge to others, they know how to do things, and new information can be more easily assimilated and compared critically with past experience.

Despite all this, it is true that there may be some loss of memory over time. It is often the short-term memory that is most vulnerable: you cannot remember what you had for lunch yesterday but you know who your classmates were at school — well, some of them anyway. Some people advocate eating certain foods to improve, or at least retain, memory. It is suggested that oily fish, fruit and vegetables, particularly those that have a lot of colour such as blueberries, beetroot, carrots and broccoli can be beneficial. Incidentally, these same foods are beneficial for many aspects of healthy living, especially those fruits and vegetables that have purple, blue or dark green colouring. These are high in antioxidants. Even when you eat may be important; there have been studies suggesting that breakfast is an essential meal for good memory performance.

Get the shots

Influenza vaccination is free for those over 65 and for people with certain chronic conditions that render them at risk of complications if they contract influenza. It is not often realised that influenza, or rather its complications, can be a major cause of serious illness and death. Getting vaccinated is a way of avoiding these problems. The procedure is simple, virtually painless and protection against current strains of the influenza virus is very good.

Dine in style

One of the most important aspects of growing older is to preserve a healthy diet. Many older people admitted to hospital suffer from some degree of malnutrition. If they need surgery, for example, they sometimes have to be fed properly beforehand. This reduces the complication rate and hastens recovery.

You might well eat smaller meals as you grow older but that should not mean that you eat inadequate meals. You still need a balanced diet with plenty of vegetables as well as animal protein, unless you are a vegetarian of course.

Many single older people do not eat properly because they cannot be bothered to cook proper meals for themselves. Also, supermarkets do not always provide smaller packages of meat or vegetables, making it more difficult for the older person to shop effectively. Already the importance of some fruits and vegetables, along with fish, has been mentioned as being beneficial to health.

If you find yourself living alone, one way to solve both the problem of loneliness and the problem of nutrition is to invite someone else living alone around for dinner. Have a roast with all the trimmings, open a bottle of wine, finish with some sticky dessert — spoil yourselves. And the next week you can go round to their place and do much the same thing. Who knows, you may end up with a convivial dining club if several of you get involved.

Don't get hooked on supplements

There are often claims made about the benefits of some dietary supplements. Be cautious about these claims, and make sure you are not paying out a lot of money for something of questionable value because some of the claims made for these supplements are unsupported by hard evidence. For example, echinacea, which has been widely promoted as a cold reliever, recently has been shown to be ineffective. Any claim that such-and-such a herb or extract will prolong your life, free up your joints, improve your memory, or all of these should be regarded with the greatest scepticism. You are much better off spending your money elsewhere or saving it for a rainy day; such products are not cheap.

However, some supplements such as glucosamine for arthritis and garlic for prevention of heart attacks do seem to have a place. Take care that there is no adverse effect when taking prescription medicines.

Most people have a diet that contains perfectly adequate amounts of all the vitamins and minerals necessary for a healthy life. Any additional intake of these essential substances results in them being broken down and wasted. There are certain exceptions; for example, some older women may need calcium supplementation to prevent or treat osteoporosis, strict vegetarians may need additional vitamins. The key to all this is a balanced diet, fish at least once a week, red meat, chicken, plenty of fresh vegetables of assorted colours, cereals for fibre and as much fruit as you like. Eat like that and supplements should not be needed.

The things that can go wrong

In this section I have tried to cover some of the common health problems people may encounter as age progresses. The list is not exhaustive and the coverage is very superficial. However, I have attempted to summarise the main points. For further information your doctor or practice nurse are invaluable sources — use them. The main problems include:

▷ arthritis

▷ heart disease and stroke

▷ diabetes

▷ cancer

▷ Alzheimer's disease.

My aching bones

Rheumatics, arthritis — call it what you will — comes in two kinds: rheumatoid arthritis and osteoarthritis. Of these, rheumatoid arthritis tends to occur in younger people and will not be considered further. Osteoarthritis is what older people mostly suffer from. Any joints may be affected. Some people have problems with the small joints of the hand; others with hips, knees, shoulders and so on. Physiotherapy may help, and pain relief can be obtained with some drugs. But all drugs have side effects and so, where possible, should not be taken long term or in large quantities.

It has been suggested, in at least one study, that glucosamine taken regularly may provide reasonable relief from pain and may act to slow the degenerative process. On the other hand, the chondroitin sulphate often sold in combination with glucosamine seems to have no proven effect. You are better spending your money on the pure glucosamine. Women are particularly prone to the condition of osteoporosis, a weakening of the bones affecting the long bones in particular, but also the vertebrae, and rendering them liable to breakage. Taking a calcium supplement may help slow down the process as many older people have a less than optimum calcium intake. Vitamin D is also important but most people have an adequate vitamin D intake. Attention to a balanced diet is as important here as elsewhere.

The joints need changing

Three joints commonly need replacement: shoulder, hip and knee. Of these, hip joint replacement is the most common and is usually undertaken on people over the age of 50. The main indication for joint replacement is pain or loss of mobility, usually both. The pain of an arthritic major joint can be severe, constant, and crippling to the extent that it affects the whole of your life. This is not the place to fully explore the problems of arthritic joints, but certainly hip replacement is mostly successful, relieves the pain, restores mobility and lasts for many years, probably the rest of your life. The operation is a major one in terms of the trauma, and recovery generally takes an initial six weeks followed by several more weeks of rehabilitation. This rehabilitation period is needed because the muscles have become weakened during the time when the joint was deteriorating and those muscles need to regain their strength. However, most people with hip replacements are reasonably active after two to three months. The recovery time after knee and shoulder replacements seem to be a bit longer but the end result is most satisfactory.

Beware of too much pressure

High blood pressure is quite common among older people and, if left untreated, can lead to all sorts of health problems. Raised blood pressure is often picked up during a routine health check or when you see the doctor for something else. It may be a sign that something else is wrong and will probably need some investigations. Once the diagnosis is made, treatment can be very effective.

Both sexes are liable to coronary artery disease and cerebrovascular disease. These may lead to heart attacks and strokes, respectively. Smoking and obesity are particular risk factors for these diseases so that stopping smoking and controlling weight are important health measures. People with raised cholesterol levels are at risk of both heart attacks and strokes. There is some evidence that your genes can also play a part. What your close blood relatives died of can be an important predictor of your own risk of heart disease. This means that if, for example, your father and your mother both died at a relatively young age of either a heart attack or a stroke, you may have a significantly increased risk of suffering the same fate. However, with newer medication, the use of daily aspirin or similar drugs, drugs for the control of high blood pressure and raised cholesterol levels the risk can be reduced quite markedly.

Get checked out

Whatever your family history, once you have passed the age of 60 it is wise to have an annual, or more frequent, check of your cholesterol levels, and a session with your family doctor. If you have had a heart attack, it does not mean that you are finished with. Modern medicine and surgery can provide you with a normal life, probably for many years. There are a number of places to seek advice, the Heart Foundation being an excellent source of good information, as well as your family doctor and specialist.

Stroke

Minor strokes, like heart attacks, affect many people over the age of 60 and some younger than that. Indeed, heart disease and stroke are the leading causes of death for older people, with stroke being a major cause for women over 85. A stroke, like a heart attack, is not the end of the world. The majority of strokes result in little or no loss of function, while more severe strokes may leave one with a weakness on one side, perhaps a limp. Major strokes resulting in speech defects and complete paralysis on one side may require a long period of rehabilitation. Obviously your life will be affected but you may still be able to enjoy many things. Measures to prevent stroke are the same as those for heart disease.

Diabetes

Type 2 diabetes may affect quite a number of older people, often those who are a bit overweight. The condition, if left untreated, can lead to kidney failure, increased risk of heart disease, and even blindness. It is the result of an imbalance between blood sugar levels and the amount of insulin produced; treatment is effective if followed strictly, and regular checks by your doctor are important. There are now available devices that allow you to measure your own blood sugar at home. With good control of your sugar levels you can expect to live a normal life.

Cancer

A word that most people dread, but cancers come in many forms, affecting different organs. Many can be successfully treated. However, treatment does not always fully cure the disease and cancer is probably the second most common cause of death in older people. Women are more prone to breast cancer and there is a good national screening programme that is free to women between the ages of 45 and 69 inclusive. For men, the most common cancers are lung, colon and prostate, but although screening tests are available there is as yet no national programme.

Many cancers, if detected very early, can be treated successfully by surgery, chemotherapy or radiotherapy, or combinations of these. As with most other diseases the knowledge that you have, or have had, a cancer is not the end of the world. Much of the remainder of your life will be dependent on your attitude to your health and to your well-being. Have a negative attitude and probably you will not live long, and you will have a poor time of it. A positive attitude, on the other hand, while it may lead to only a small prolongation of life, will certainly make that life so much more enjoyable for yourself and for those around you.

Problems with the mind

Alzheimer's disease is probably the best known of the dementias that afflict some older people. Alzheimer's disease itself is a serious cause of major memory loss and bizarre behaviour affecting a small number of older people, although the disease sometimes strikes much younger people. While the overall progress of the disease at present cannot be halted, there are several steps that make the tragic journey from first symptoms to death more bearable for both the sufferer and their loved ones.

Help should be sought at the first signs of real and significant memory loss. There are now memory clinics being set up that can assist and help slow down the progress of the disease, and an early diagnosis can lead to some improvement and initiate support for the family. There also are drugs under development that may slow down memory loss.

Depression has already been mentioned in the section on relationships (see page 41). A surprising number of older people do suffer from minor, or major, depression and the condition may not be apparent to friends and family. It is up to all of us to be aware of the problem and to try and recognise that someone is seriously down in the dumps and in need of treatment.

Stress

Much is said about stress these days. It is very easy to say 'I feel stressed out' when the slightest problem presents itself. Get a grip! Some stress is probably good for you. It improves performance and keeps you sharp. If there's a problem deal with it or ask someone who can help. Do not let yourself slide into incessant worry over things that can be sorted — sort them.

It's not all gloomy

Health can always be a depressing subject but we should

not let it be filled with gloom. There are many positive aspects of health, not least the good news when you have been successfully treated and given a new warrant of fitness. By being positive about health, being sensible about one's limitations, and getting the problems attended to while they are still minor, we can all hope to enjoy the good life for that much longer.

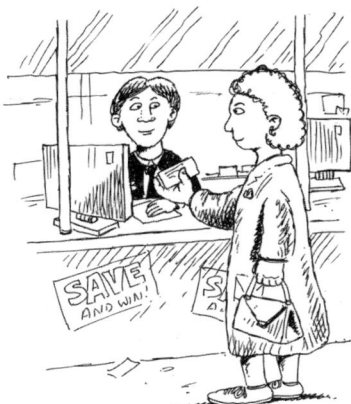

9

Money matters

Financial planning

Money does matter. It is not possible to think about retirement without considering the cost of living and the need for an adequate income. The New Zealand superannuation is set at a fairly low percentage of the average wage and will not buy you very much. It goes without saying that some sort of saving for retirement is essential if you are going to be able to enjoy the third age. It has been said before: if you retire at 65 in good health you can expect to have as long as 20 years of life or more remaining. Twenty years is a long time and, although financial needs usually decrease with advancing age, you will still need to have your enhanced income over the whole of that time. The time to start saving for retirement is when one first starts earning. Most people will not do this. Many will not even have started by the time they are 40. It really is never too early to start.

Stock up while you can

If you have a substantial garden, or will be moving to one, take care to buy all your likely machinery needs ahead of your retirement time. Most machinery, lawnmowers, hedge trimmers, chainsaws and so on, will have a life of about ten years. To start buying this equipment when your income is reduced will hurt. Do it before you stop earning. The same applies to whiteware, televisions; any appliance that will be expensive to replace. Replacement ahead of time will save you money and anguish in the longer term. Indeed, any object or property that you believe will be an essential component of your retirement should be acquired before you stop work.

Becoming a pensioner

When you reach 65 you will be entitled to New Zealand superannuation for which you need to apply to Work and Income New Zealand (WINZ). The WINZ case officer at the first interview should take you through the pension benefits to which you are entitled; make sure this is done. The benefits will depend on your marital status and the age of your partner, along with your tax status.

The case officer should also explain to you the additional benefits to which you may be entitled: such as an accommodation allowance, a special needs grant, a living alone payment and several others relating to health, emergencies and housing. Unfortunately, there are some older people missing out on benefits they could be receiving. One reason for this is that they may not have fully understood, or not been listening to, the things that have been said to them, or provided in written material. Families are important here in helping their ageing relatives understand the options.

Planning for saving

There are a number of publications available that provide advice on saving for retirement. Among the most comprehensive is the series of brochure-type publications issued by the Retirement Commission. These cover much the same ground as some older, but now out of print, Consumers' Institute publications but in a more compact form. This information is available on the Retirement Commission's website (see page 122).

Pay it all off

The first place to start is to get rid of debt, or at least minimise it. By the time you reach retirement you should be absolutely debt free. This is an important savings mechanism and one often neglected by otherwise sensible people. Once you have got rid of debt, which includes mortgage, you can call your money your own and spend or invest it as you choose.

How much will you need?

Most people over the age of 65 in New Zealand, whether single or as couples, do not have very substantial incomes. Information from the Ministry of Social Policy puts the median net annual income for single people at $12,090 and at $21,000 for couples. Three-quarters of single people in 2001 had an annual income of under $15,300 and three-quarters of couples had an income under $32,500.

These income levels result in many individuals and couples living a life that is filled with anxieties, cheap cuts of meat, second-hand clothes, poorly heated houses, and so on. Their standard of well-being may be quite low. These people have little or nothing to fall back on and it is no surprise to learn that the biggest headaches come when a major item, a washing machine or an oven for instance, has to be replaced, or there is an unexpectedly large repair bill for the car.

On the other hand information from the Ministry suggests that 39 percent of people over the age of 65 have a material well-being score that is average for this age group, and that although there are some restrictions on such things as the frequency of holidays, or overseas visits, they can manage fairly well on a limited income. These people did not get there without some planning because in all instances they have an income level that is quite a lot higher than that provided by New Zealand superannuation.

So what is the lower limit for a really comfortable income after retirement? Of course, there is no complete answer because one person's limit may be much lower than another's. Although we all have much the same needs we all have different wants! It all depends on the lifestyle choice, given good health. With poor health and limited mobility the limit may be quite a lot lower unless payment for health care is a concern. A useful guide is that you should aim for a total income that is about 70 percent of your final salary or wage. If you are now 40 or so just work on 70 percent of what you currently earn and add a bit to that.

Working out what saving you have to do in order to have the income you want is quite easy. The Retirement Commission's website includes an online calculator, as do the websites of several banks. Unless you are quite young the results you get are not pretty! You really do have to save quite a lot of money once you reach the age of 40 if you want to have anything like a decent post-retirement income.

How to save

There are several ways of saving for retirement, some better or safer than others, but all should be considered and ideally more than one mechanism for saving should be adopted. The various savings options are only broadly discussed here; they are more fully described in a number of books as well as in the publications mentioned previously. This section can also be considered as an aid to the investment of any substantial funds you may have at the time of retirement to provide income over subsequent years.

Get the best advice

A number of books and magazines recommend that you seek the advice of a financial adviser before investing whatever you have saved, and many people undoubtedly benefit from the advice of someone experienced in finance. There are a number of extremely reputable and reliable financial advisers, but there also are a few dodgy ones. Be aware that many advisers get paid twice. Not only do you pay for their services, but also they may be paid a commission, or get a free trip or two, or be rewarded in some similar way, for pushing your business towards a specific financial product. There are some advisers who are fully independent and will receive only payment from the client. If you do want the services of somebody to help you with investment, try to ensure that the person you choose is truly independent; that is, is not linked to a specific financial management group. In this way you can be confident of getting advice that is objective and unbiased.

Professional regulation

The Financial Planners and Insurance Advisers Association tries to ensure that members fully disclose any commission or other benefit they gain from recommending particular financial products. The association has a code of conduct and a disciplinary process. However, while it is compulsory in New Zealand for advisers to disclose any convictions involving dishonesty and any instances where they have been banned from participating in the management of a company or business, there is at present no requirement to disclose what qualifications and experience the adviser has or what commissions the adviser might receive. So make sure that the adviser you use is a member of that association, and do ask about qualifications, experience in the industry and any commission the adviser might get.

Managed funds

A managed fund is an investment vehicle whereby the contributions of all its investors are pooled and a manager, acting according to the mandate of the fund, invests in a diverse variety of investments that may include shares, bonds, fixed interest and so on. There are four main types of managed funds in New Zealand:

▷ superannuation funds

▷ unit trusts

▷ group investment funds

▷ insurance bonds.

There are differences in legal issues, tax, and ownership between these four types of funds, differences that may influence your choice depending on your tax status and financial objectives. Each of these funds is described below.

All managed funds provide an investment statement, a document that provides all the details you are likely to need. An investment statement will include:

▷ the country of investment

▷ what the fee structure is

▷ type of investment; for example, insurance bond, superannuation fund

▷ the sorts of assets the fund holds; for example, share, bonds

▷ the tax structure

▷ projected future returns

▷ the risks involved

▷ administrative information

▷ an application form.

Fees, fees, fees

One problem with managed funds is the fee structure. It seems that many funds have a fee structure that is not in the best interests of investors. The fees charged can eat up much, if not all, of the returns of the fund. At the time of writing there has been further criticism of the fees charged, particularly by balanced funds. The Consumers' Institute (*Consumer*, June 2004) issued figures suggesting that people would have been better off putting their money in a savings account over a ten-year period. Not surprisingly, the investment industry has criticised the criticism and attempted to defend its position. The message in all of this is to examine the fee structure carefully and make your decision based on firm facts rather than on promises of future high returns. This issue is discussed further below.

Employer pension schemes

There was a time when almost every large employer had a compulsory contributory pension scheme. The employee paid in so much a week or month and that was matched by some contribution from the employer. At retirement workers were guaranteed a fairly high percentage of their final salary or wage, a scheme called 'defined benefit'. The recent trend has been to move away from that type of scheme to the 'defined contribution' scheme, where the final payment is dependent on the market or markets in which the funds are invested. In essence the defined contribution scheme is little different from the commercial superannuation savings schemes available and subject to the same advantages and disadvantages (see below).

If your employer does have a subsidised superannuation scheme you will probably, if not certainly, be a contributor. Such schemes are very worthwhile and the savings gained can exceed those resulting from paying off a mortgage. It is one instance when paying off the debt should be delayed. It is likely that such a scheme will have 'vesting' rules, whereby you must remain a contributor to the scheme for a set period, usually five to ten years, before you are entitled to the employer's contribution as well as your own. The State Services Retirement Scheme, introduced in 2004, seems to be a good model for future schemes.

Even if the employer does not match your own contributions there are additional benefits if the employer pays the fees of the fund as these can amount to several hundred dollars over the years. In a pamphlet on investing the Retirement Commission gives an example:

A man chose to pay into a commercial superannuation fund instead of the one offered by his employer who would have paid the fees. The difference in savings over a three-year period would have been $700, the amount of the fees.

Certainly, if you are going to be with the same employer

for a significant time and an employer-backed, fees-paid scheme is available it provides an excellent way of saving.

Many employers now seem to have opted out of pension schemes. Indeed, few employers seem to take any interest in the futures of those who are retiring, although several years ago many firms had pre-retirement education programmes along with their pension schemes.

Where to put the money

Whether you are saving for retirement, or wanting to invest a sum you have saved once you retire, you will need to have an investment strategy. This strategy will determine:

> ▷ what sort of returns you hope to receive

> ▷ what sort of investments you are going to make

> ▷ how much you are going to place in each of these

> ▷ the location of your investments, in New Zealand or overseas.

Some of the investment opportunities that exist are considered below. This book cannot advise you about which to choose because everybody's situation is different. If you want that kind of advice carefully choose a financial adviser and follow, or choose not to follow, their advice.

Commercial superannuation funds

These are funds established to assist you in saving for retirement. You pay in so much each month, or more frequently, and that money is invested on your behalf in a variety of investment instruments, commonly fixed interest deposits, bonds and so on. There are two types of superannuation funds: locked and unlocked. A locked fund requires you to keep all your funds 'locked' in the fund until a certain time has elapsed. Some such funds do allow a small proportion of your funds to be withdrawn annually, but usually only after you have been paying into the fund for some time.

Unlocked funds, on the other hand, allow you to withdraw your savings at any time. Unlocked funds are sometimes considered superior because the manager has a greater incentive to provide a good return on your investment so that you do not take your money elsewhere. However, locked funds may have lower fees. Before you decide on either of these investment options you should consider what your returns over time might be with alternative investments such as unit trusts, group investment funds (GIFs), bonds, shares, or even cash, as well as getting more information on each of the funds.

Fees again

Again, you should pay particular attention to fees when choosing one of these funds. Some schemes charge an entry fee that can be a percentage of each contribution, and also an exit fee when you withdraw your savings. In addition, funds usually charge an ongoing monthly fee for managing the fund. Fair enough, but check on the size of this fee as it can affect your savings; it may be as much as 1.5 percent per year, although many funds charge a monthly fee. Funds may also charge an annual 'policy' fee, while some also run a two-tier system whereby, for a period of up to two years your initial deposits go into a 'foundation' account, or purchase 'initial units'. Only when you have made these investments does your money start to go into the investment account. The problem with this is that the fees on these initial investments are often as much as 5 percent and that can apply for the whole term of your investment.

Many funds quote their fees in percentage terms. If you are looking for a fund ask for the fees to be quoted in dollar terms. Many fund managers will not agree to do this but it does no harm to ask. If you receive a negative answer, perhaps you should take your investment elsewhere.

Most managed funds have an entry fee, an exit fee, a management fee, an annual Management Expense Ratio (MER, calculated on the total value of the fund) and an annual trustees fee. If there are more fees than these, if the fee structure looks complicated, or if there is a two-tier system, walk away and look elsewhere. Fees can seriously affect your investment and mean you may not be getting as much as you thought, or even as much as you should.

Good years and bad years
Most of these superannuation funds have good years when the fund makes a profit, and bad years when the fund makes a loss. You should be aware of this before you start investing. Just because last year a particular fund returned, say, 9 percent on investment does not mean that it is a hot potato; it may be a lemon and fall to −2 percent next year. Get the historical earnings of any fund you are thinking of; one place to look is the Fund Source website (see page 126). This site, which is free to join, provides data on a large number of managed funds of all types. It also has its own grading system for funds and provides a star rating, five being very good, one being poor.

Unit trusts
Unit trusts are a type of managed fund in which the pooled contributions of investors, who purchase 'units', are used to invest in a variety of investments. Unit trusts have a trustee who administers the trust deed, which specifies how

the trust is managed and what it can invest in. The trustee makes sure that the manager, who does the day-to-day work, performs in accordance with the trust deed.

Investment is usually by lump sum but many trusts have a savings facility whereby monthly, or fortnightly, regular savings can be made, usually $100 or more. Unit trusts pay dividends called 'distributions', which can, if you wish, be used to purchase additional units: a good way of increasing your investment. Alternatively, if you have invested after retirement, the distributions can be an additional source of income, perhaps even your major source.

Group investment funds

These are similar to unit trusts and are usually provided by trustee companies with the fund manager acting as the trustee. Many GIFs invest in mortgages and low-risk investments, but several are more diversified with investment in equities. Some are 'index' funds, which passively track a particular share index such as the NZ 50, although most are still on the NZ 40 index. A passive investment such as this should mirror the index it is based on in terms of values and dividends. The management fees for index-linked funds are generally lower than for active funds as the manager has less of a decision-making role.

Insurance bonds

Insurance bonds, managed by insurance companies and some banks, are also similar to unit trusts but they are taxed before any distribution reaches you. The company pays tax on any profits at 33 percent. Like unit trusts and GIFs, insurance bonds are unitised and the exit price of units is usually quoted in the newspapers. Fees may be lower than for some other managed funds.

Investment trusts

These are companies that pool money and buy shares. They are quoted on the share market and shares in the trusts can be bought and sold through a share broker, who will charge brokerage. Unlike unit trusts, investment trusts can borrow to buy shares, a process known as 'gearing'. A large number of these trusts are based overseas, but several are traded on the New Zealand market. Because the shares are similar to shares in a company, there is no complicated fee structure, and any fees are based on the total asset value, not on your own investment. One of the advantages of investment trusts is that the price of their shares may be lower than the price of the constituent shares on the market. Of course, the price may also be higher, reflecting optimism that the price of the underlying shares is going to rise.

Shares

Investment in shares can be a major part of the investment strategy of prudent investors. Shares are not for everyone, and there is always a greater element of risk than with some other investments. However, with thought and discipline, a portfolio of shares can be very rewarding.

Shares are portions of a company's 'equity'; that is, the amount paid by the owners of the company to establish it. Companies may also raise money by borrowing, or by the issue of further shares. Each share then represents a part of that company's capital. Shares usually can be traded on the share market and may increase or decrease in value over time. Usually, but not always, the company will pay a dividend, part of the company's profit, on each share annually or half-yearly. This dividend sometimes can be used to purchase additional shares in the company, but usually is paid to you directly. If you hold sufficient shares in a company, or companies, the dividends you get will be an additional source of income, and some retirees rely heavily on shares for this purpose.

Shares are of several kinds. 'Ordinary' shares carry voting rights, which means the shareholder can attend any shareholder meeting and vote on any proposed changes in company policy. The shareholders also elect the board of directors of the company.

Find a broker
Shares are purchased through a broker, who is a member of the New Zealand Stock Exchange (NZSX) and who will charge a small percentage of the transaction as a fee. Shares are usually bought in sizeable lots. A $5 note will not get you far, so if you have limited funds you are better off investing in shares through some sort of managed fund.

What colour are your chips?
Companies come and go; some are very long lived and continue to prosper — they are regarded as solid, or 'blue chip' shares. Any portfolio should be composed of shares in several blue chip companies. Ideally, a share portfolio needs to be diversified — made up of shares in a variety of industries. In this way risk can be reduced because different industries rarely all do badly at the same time.

Shares are for those who can afford to be in for the long haul. Over the short term, shares can fluctuate quite markedly in value, but the overall trend for good-quality stock will be to increase in value over time. This is what happens to the market overall, this is what investors are looking for, and this is why you have to be prepared to hold onto your shares through the troughs and the peaks in value. If you are constantly in and out of the market, buying and selling shares aggressively, you may become liable to tax on any capital gains that you make because you are regarded as trading. However, if you sell your shares only after holding them for a long time you probably will not be liable to capital gains tax; another reason for holding on.

Keeping a close eye on performance

Of course, you will want to keep an eye on your investments; share prices are quoted in the financial pages of daily papers. Several bits of information are provided for each share: the closing buy and sell offer prices, the share price high and low over the past year, dividends paid in cents per share, yield, the dividend as a percentage of the current share price, profit/earnings ratio, a ratio between the market price and the earnings per share, whether the share is ex-dividend, and so on. There are also some software packages that enable you to keep track of your share prices over a longer period of time. These often come with fancy graph capabilities that can be fun for those so minded and enable the sophisticated kind of analysis that the professionals use.

Property

For most people their house is their biggest asset; however, it brings in no money. Indeed, it costs you money in insurance, rates and maintenance. The only way you can realise the cash tied up in your house is by selling it; only then you will have nowhere to live! There is another option. There are now available 'Reverse Equity Mortgages' (RAMs) or 'Home Equity Release' (HER) schemes. These enable you to borrow against a percentage of the equity in your house and either receive a lump sum or a fortnightly or monthly annuity payment. You pay interest and any set-up fees at maturity so that you are not making regular mortgage payments. One company will lend 10 percent of the property value to 60–64 year olds, with a 5 percent increase for every age group step. At age 90 you can borrow 40 percent of the value of your property. There are other companies offering similar schemes with differences only in interest rates, eligibility and set-up fees. At least one of the schemes allows you to transfer the loan to another property if you decide to move, provided that the equity proportion is maintained.

Such schemes are attractive if you do not need to leave the whole of the equity tied up in your property to your children. Also, if you live to the end of the loan period there may not be much left after the compound interest has been added to the original loan; another example of there being no such thing as a free lunch. Increasingly, however, children do not have the expectation that they will inherit bags of money from their parents' estate, and many would rather their parents had an enjoyable lifestyle as they grow older. This is not to say that a RAM or HER is right for everyone. If you think such an idea is attractive, you should certainly discuss it with your family and your solicitor.

Become a landlord

Many people purchase property additional to their family home and rent the property out to provide them with an income. On the other hand, they may make some improvements to the building and sell it on at a profit. Most property investors choose the first of these. They may end up owning several houses that they rent out. It is likely that many of these people needed to borrow in order to buy their properties, but that is no problem provided the rental income more than meets the mortgage payments plus property maintenance, rates and insurance.

Is residential property investment still a worthwhile

strategy? Residential property prices have risen considerably in the past few years, particularly in the Auckland region. It is becoming harder to find suitable properties for investment. Nevertheless, there may well be opportunities in several locations for residential property investment.

Before you decide to get into residential property investment you should be aware that planning is all important. Conservative budgeting, taking into account the fact that tenants do not last for ever and you may have a month or more without rent coming in each year, will reveal whether or not you can snaffle up that house round the corner. Bear in mind that owning one or more houses for rent means that you will have to spend quite a bit of time looking after your business. You, as the landlord, will have to deal with tenants, respond to maintenance requests, keep track of rental payments and so on. Some people put their properties in the hands of a property management company, often itself a real estate agency.

Cash

Ideally, you should always keep some of your investment funds in some sort of savings fund where the money is readily accessible. Savings funds, available at trading banks, savings banks and most finance companies, do not pay huge amounts of interest, but they all pay some interest and your money can continue to grow. To make sure it does grow at the best rate make sure that the bank or finance company calculates and pays interest at regular intervals.

There is no agreed percentage of funds that should be kept this way, but if your total sum available for investment is quite modest you should consider putting most of the money into an interest-bearing account.

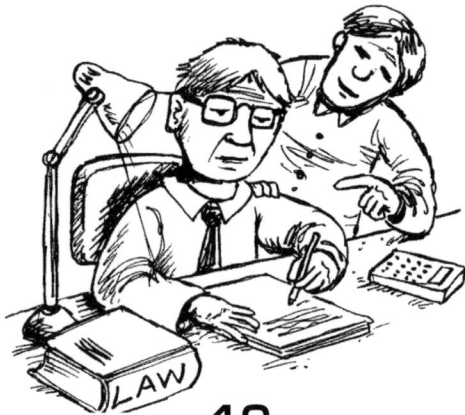

10

Getting things straight

Legal matters

There are a number of situations in which you may benefit from the advice or services of a lawyer, but you can save yourself quite a bit of bother by first consulting one of the many pamphlets put out by the New Zealand Law Society. These cover a variety of topics, including: the implications of recent legislation covering the sharing of assets when relationships break down, making a will, family trusts, buying and selling property and so on. All the pamphlets are available either from the society or from one of the district law societies.

This section deals with some of the legal matters that are especially likely to concern those in, or near, the third age.

Family trusts

The possibility of becoming too frail to live in one's own home and having to realise assets in order to pay for a rest home bed has led to many people forming a family trust. There may, of course, be other reasons for forming such trusts but asset protection usually is a large component of the decision. Forming a family trust should not be an expensive process. However, some lawyers and accountants seem to regard family trusts as a nice little earner and charge quite high fees so it pays to shop around. There are normally two kinds of fees: a setting-up fee and an annual fee for processing the gifting of assets through the Inland Revenue Department. Some firms may charge an additional fee for acting as a trustee.

Asset protection sounds like a good idea and it probably is under the present rules. But there is nothing to prevent some greedy government in the future from legislating to block asset protection. It is unlikely to happen in the near future because many politicians have their own family trusts!

There are two main kinds of trusts. The first is a trust that contains only specified assets, usually the family property, but can also include valuable assets such as art, antique furniture, rare books, old motor cars and so on. The second kind of trust may include sources of income in addition to assets, with the ability to share that income among the various beneficiaries. The income may derive from assets such as shares or rental properties.

Trustees are usually three in number, but may be fewer. For many family trusts the trustees are usually husband and wife and a third trustee, who may be a lawyer or accountant, or even a friend.

Making a will

Even if you have not yet retired you should have made a will. A will is not irrevocable; it can be changed, ripped up, revised, rewritten, but only by you! Some lawyers and trustee companies do not charge for drawing up a will if they are to be the executors, but many will charge a small fee, about $100. You can get do-it-yourself blank will forms from some larger bookshops, but the recommendation is that the final document be discussed with a lawyer or trustee company. Your will should cover how you wish your assets to be distributed, what specific bequests you wish to make, who your executor will be, how you wish your body disposed of and how funeral costs are to be met. These last may come out of your estate, but many people now have pre-paid funeral plans – a good idea.

The executor

As you get older the place of a will in your life becomes more important. There will usually be a surviving partner to look after, and children and grandchildren you may wish to benefit in some way. There may be heirlooms, family portraits, rare books, art, an old car or whatever, that you wish to leave to specific people. In choosing an executor, the person, or persons, who will administer your estate and see that your wishes are carried out, you will need to consider any fees involved.

Lawyers and trustee companies will charge a fee based either on an hourly rate for the work or a percentage of the value of the estate. The former is likely to be much cheaper; for a $300,000 estate trustee companies may charge up to $10,000. However, if you make one or more family members, or someone else whom you trust as your executors there will usually be no cost involved. Be certain, however, that you fully trust whomever you choose to carry out your wishes to the full and without bias. It probably also helps to choose as an executor someone in good health with a likelihood of surviving you! If you choose a family member it could be wise to choose two who would act as co-executors.

The executor will: make sure that the body is disposed of in accordance with the will; obtain assets and settle debts; pay any tax; establish any trusts to be set up under the will; obtain probate, usually done by a lawyer; distribute the estate. Because these tasks may be quite complex many people prefer to leave the whole business of being an executor to the family lawyer.

Powers of attorney

Powers of attorney are documents that give someone else the power to act on your behalf when you cannot act yourself. These documents can limit the actions to what may, and may not, be done.

There are two kinds of power of attorney: 'ordinary' and 'enduring'. The former is used for a limited period of time and operates only while you are mentally competent; it lapses should you become mentally incompetent. It is the sort of thing you might wish to use if you are going on an overseas trip, for example, to ensure that the bills are paid and other affairs managed.

Ordinary power of attorney

As mentioned above this is the sort of power that you formally give to someone to manage some or all of your affairs while you are overseas or perhaps in hospital and unable to take direct action yourself. You can be quite specific about the affairs you wish to have managed, and you can even appoint more than one attorney. If you do this you can specify whether they must act jointly or separately ('severally' in legal terms). You might, for instance, appoint one person to manage your bank account and pay the bills, and another to let out your house while you are away.

You can create an ordinary power of attorney only while you are legally competent; that is, you have the physical and mental capacity to provide instructions. As soon as you become mentally incompetent the ordinary power of attorney ceases to exist. Also, you cannot convert your ordinary power of attorney into an enduring power of attorney. In general, the ordinary power of attorney also ceases if you die, with the powers passing to the executor(s) of your will.

To create an ordinary power of attorney you need to complete a standard form that is available from lawyers, trustee companies and some stationers. In the form you specify what powers you are giving to your attorney and whether the power is time limited or open ended.

Enduring power of attorney

Enduring power of attorney is something everyone in retirement should have and is drawn up in such a way that it comes into operation once you are no longer able to manage your own affairs. Enduring powers of attorney are used to either look after your property or arrange for your personal care and welfare; for each of these there will be a separate document. Because of the legal issues involved, the whole thing should be set up through a lawyer or trustee company. Usually you would appoint your partner or some other family member as attorney for each of these functions, but sometimes it might be more desirable for the property side of things to appoint two people to act 'jointly, but not severally', meaning neither can act alone and both must agree on any action. You should be aware that trustee companies will not take on the 'personal care and welfare' power, and also that any professionals you use will charge for their services.

By the time your faculties are beginning to dim it is really too late to act. Set up your powers of attorney while you are still in full command of your affairs; and this applies to your partner as well. It is a sad fact that some relatives misuse their powers as attorneys to the disadvantage of a vulnerable individual and other family members. If there is any doubt at all about the people you would choose to represent your best interests, appoint a family lawyer as your attorney.

The advance directive

Another document you may wish to draw up well ahead of time is an 'advance directive' that specifies certain actions to be taken, or not taken, in the event of serious and life–threatening surgical or medical conditions. An advanced directive may, for instance, direct that you should be allowed to die peacefully without being hooked up to life support equipment in the event that you are no longer capable of independent existence. Your family doctor and family lawyer will be able to help with this document.

Want more?

Further information and useful addresses

This section does not seek to be all inclusive. A selection of government departments and national organisations is about all that can be given as each locality has its own clubs, societies and interest groups. While some of these are listed in local telephone directories, many are not; in which case the Citizens Advice Bureau or the local library may be able to help. All government departments and their websites are listed in the telephone book — admittedly in small print!

Some bedtime reading
easypcprojects, Richard Wentk, British Consumers' Association, 2003. Available from the Consumers' Institute of New Zealand

General stuff
The Retirement Commission
PO Box 12 148, Wellington
Tel: 0800 438 767 or 04 499 7396
Fax: 04 4997397
Email: office@sorted.org.nz
Website: www.sorted.org.nz

Consumers' Institute of New Zealand Inc.
Private Bag 6996, 39 Webb St, Wellington 6035
Tel: 04 384 7963, Fax: 04 385 8752
Email: chiefexec@consumer.org.nz
Website: www.consumer.org.nz

Age Concern New Zealand
PO Box 10 688, Wellington
Tel: 04 471 2709
Fax: 04 473 2504
Email: national.office@ageconcern.org.nz
Website: www.ageconcern.org.nz
Local Age Concern councils are listed in the white
pages of the telephone book

Grey Power
www.greypower.co.nz

Citizens Advice Bureau
Call free: 0800 367 222
Website: www.cab.org.nz
Local bureaus are listed in the white pages of the
telephone book

Legal stuff
The New Zealand Law Society
P.O. Box 5041, Wellington
Tel: 04 472 7837
Fax: 04 915 1285
Website: www.nzls.org.nz
District law societies are listed in the white pages of
the telephone book

Public Trust
Website: www.publictrust.co.nz
Local branches are listed in the white pages of the
telephone directory

Where to live

Eldernet
Website: www.eldernet.co.nz

Retirement villages
www.retirementvillages.org.nz
www.fullmoon.co.nz

Learning stuff

Many educational institutions have their own websites, a few of which are listed here. Information is available also through local telephone directories, while newspapers sometimes have details of courses.

Universities
www.auckland.ac.nz
www.canterbury.ac.nz
www.massey.ac.nz
www.otago.ac.nz
www.vuw.ac.nz
www.waikato.ac.nz

Polytechnics
These can be accessed through a single website:
www.itpnz.ac.nz

University of the Third Age
www3.griffith.edu.au has a directory of most U3A groups in Australia and New Zealand, with links to other U3A services

Seniornet
Seniornet groups have courses on computer use taught by seniors:
www.seniornet.org.nz

Local groups are listed in the white pages of the telephone book

Libraries and books
www.libraries.org.nz — a directory of most public libraries that enables book searches; it can usually be used at your local library

Some search engines
www.altavista.com
www.ask.com
www.google.com
www.yahoo.com

Keeping well: health and fitness stuff
Sports and recreation
www.sparc.org.nz
Information on fitness programmes and walks in New Zealand

Everybody
Website: www.everybody.co.nz
This is a useful site for health information

Weka
Website: www.weka.org.nz
A site devoted to services for people with disabilities

The National Heart Foundation of New Zealand
PO Box 17-160, Greenlane, Auckland
Tel: 09 571 9191
Website: www.heart.org.nz

The Stroke Foundation
Website: www.stroke.org.nz

Arthritis Foundation
Website: www.arthritis.org.nz

The New Zealand Cancer Society
Website: www.cancernz.org.nz
Local branches of the society are listed in the white pages of the telephone book

Alzheimer's disease
Website: www.alzheimers.co.nz (at time of writing this site is being developed)
Local Alzheimer's societies are listed in the white pages of the telephone book

Money stuff

Work and Income New Zealand (WINZ)
Tel: (superannuation) 0800 552 002
Website: www.workandincome.govt.nz
Local service centres are listed under government phone listings in the blue pages of the telephone book

Fund Source
www.fundsource.co.nz

Calculators
As well as the Retirement Commission's site (see above), some trading banks also offer savings calculators. An example is available on the National Bank's site: www.nbnz.co.nz/personal/calculators/superannuation.asp

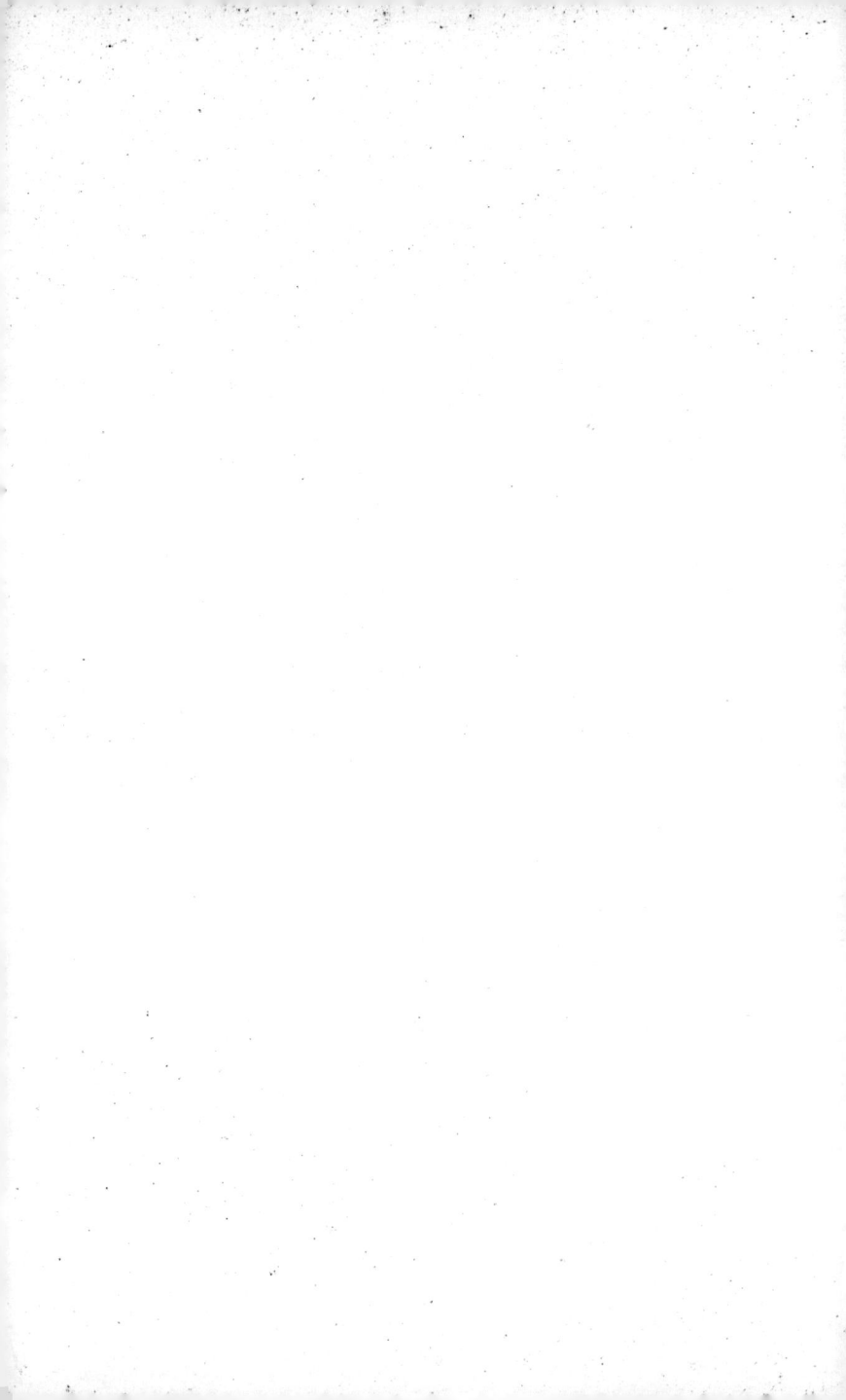